Ace the PCCN®!

You can do it!

Practice Question Review Book

Nicole Kupchik

MN, RN, CCNS, CCRN, PCCN, CMC

Nicole Kupchik Consulting, Inc.
Seattle, WA

Nicole Kupchik
P.O. Box 28053
Seattle, WA 98118

www.nicolekupchikconsulting.com

Special thanks...

To my husband, Carl

My mom, Carol

My many awesome friends
(you all know who you are...)

Dr. Elizabeth Bridges

Marilyn Richards

Karen Lynn Maher

Gina O'Daniel

My colleagues at Harborview & Swedish who have
always encouraged me over the years!

And the THOUSANDS of nurses who attended
my classes, gave constructive feedback and took the exams!
You are all an inspiration to me!

The encouragement you all have given me is
immeasurable and completely appreciated!

Foreword

The Institute of Medicine's landmark report the *Future of Nursing* issued a call for nurses to lead, including nursing leadership at the point of care.[1] While we often think about leadership as a position, it has another definition. **A leader is "an expert clinician, involved in providing direct clinical care, who influences others to continuously improve the care they provide."** [2]

One key aspect to providing this leadership is clinical expertise and the ability to use evidence to inform practice. Preparation for certification is more than the rote memorization of facts. It is about teasing out complex situations and identifying critical information to guide your practice. The process of preparing for certification will advance your knowledge, competence and understanding the complexities of critical care nursing. [3]

But equally important to the increase in overt knowledge, this process will have less obvious or conceptual effects, such as an increased awareness of the evidence that support your practice, an increased confidence in your ability and passion to use evidence culminating in the "aha" moments when concepts come to life. Ultimately this subtle and empowering use of evidence supports its more overt or instrumental use, to persuade others and to advocate for practice and policy change. [4][5]

How do these concepts apply to this book? *Ace the PCCN: You Can Do It!*

1   Institute of Medicine Committee on the Robert Wood Johnson Foundation Initiative on the Future of Nursing at IoM. The Future of Nursing: Leading Change, Advancing Health. Washington (DC): *National Academies Press* (US); 2011.

2   Cook MJ. Improving care requires leadership in nursing. *Nurse Educ Today*. 1999;19(4):306-12.

3   Sayre C, Wyant S, Karvonen C. Effect of a medical-surgical practice and certification review course on clinical nursing practice. *J Nurs Staff Dev.* 2010;26(1):11-6.

4   Nutley S, Walter I, Davies H. How research can inform public services. Bristol, UK: *The Policy Press,* 2007.

5   Wilkinson JE. *Impacts of evidence use-hard hitting or subtle change? Worldviews on Evidence-Based Nursing.* 2010;7(1):1-3.

is a book designed to help you gain knowledge and enhance your ability to interpret and respond to complex clinical situations. But this book is not just a resource to aid you in preparing for a certification examination. Rather it reflects the author's passion to support your development as an expert progressive care nurse. Along the way, the process towards certification may enhance both your conceptual and instrumental use of evidence. Think back to the definition of leadership, this journey to certification is really a journey to leadership and the advancement of our profession, and that is exactly what Nicole Kupchik is committed to.

—Elizabeth Bridges
PhD, RN, CCNS, FCCM, FAAN

Unless we are making
progress in our nursing
every year, every month, every week,
take my word for it,
we are going back.

—Florence Nightingale (May 1872)

Contents

A note of encouragement from Nicole...

Congratulations on taking steps to becoming certified and obtaining the PCCN®!

In 2002, I passed the CCRN® for the first time. I am going to let you in on a little secret. I was eligible to sit the exam in 1994. I attended three certification review courses before taking the exam. Why? I lacked confidence and was so afraid of failing. I finally got up the courage in 2002 and aced it!

I can distinctly remember walking out of the testing site questioning myself and why I waited so long to take it. I had so much self-doubt. It was a little crazy, because clinically, I knew my stuff. A couple years later I started teaching sections of the exam at Harborview and in 2006 started co-teaching the prep courses nationally.

Who would think someone could go from having a complete lack of confidence to teaching the courses a few years later? Mental mindset is everything! I want you to tell yourself every day that you can do this!!!

I often hear nurses say "becoming certified doesn't make you a better nurse". I completely disagree with statements like that. The journey you will take in preparing to become certified increases your knowledge to better care for your patients. I truly believe every nurse should be certified in their specialty.

I was inspired to publish this book by nurses who attended my review courses. Many of the study books available are overwhelming & contain too much information. My goal is always to break down disease states into digestible pieces so you learn.

My biggest piece of advice to you in studying is, of course to understand different conditions, but do as many practice test questions as possible. Read rationales for questions you get right & those you miss. Consider using *Ace the PCCN®: You can do it! Study Guide* to assist. The book was written in an easy to read format with bullet pointed content. I believe practicing questions and understanding the content is the key to success!

You can do it!

About the Contributors

Michelle A. Dedeo DNP, RN, CNS, ACCNS-AG, CCRN

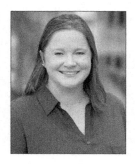

Michelle received her Bachelor of Science in Nursing from the University of Wisconsin Madison and her Masters in Nursing and Doctorate in Nursing Practice from the University of Washington. She works for Legacy Health and teaches for Linfield College, both in Portland, OR.

James "Charlie" Edwards BSN, RN, CCRN, CEN

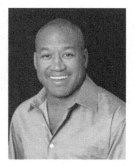

James "Charlie" Edwards earned his Bachelor of Science in Nursing from the University of Phoenix and is pursuing a Masters in Nursing from Western Governors University (projected graduation February 2017). He has been a nurse for over 25 years and is currently the Clinical Educator for Critical Care Services/Cardiac Cath Lab/Interventional Radiology at Desert Regional Medical Center in Palm Springs, California.

Toufic S. Khairallah MSN, APN, FNP-BC, PCCN, CHSE

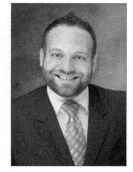

Toufic S. Khairallah (T.K.) is a board-certified Family Nurse Practitioner with a background as an RN in Cardio-Thoracic Progressive and Critical Care Services. He became a clinical nurse educator in 2008. Currently he is a Clinical Education Nurse Scholar specializing in Healthcare Simulation at OSF Saint Francis Medical Center and is also a clinical medical education associate at the University of Illinois, College of Medicine at Peoria.

Kristin Nathan BSN, RN, CCRN

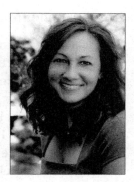

Kristin Nathan works as a clinical nurse educator in the Cardio Vascular Intensive Care Unit at Legacy Emanuel Medical Center in Portland, Oregon. She earned her Bachelor of Science in Nursing from Ohio State University and is currently pursuing her Masters in Nursing Education. She has spent the past 18 years practicing as a critical care nurse and educator in cardiovascular medicine. She has held a position as a clinical adjunct faculty at Linfield Good Samaritan School of Nursing.

Kyla F Woodward MN, RN

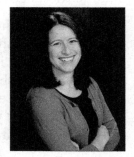

Kyla has 16 years of experience in nursing with a clinical background in trauma and surgical critical care, progressive care, and stroke. After earning her Masters in Nursing, Kyla worked as a critical and progressive care educator in the hospital setting. She has taught a variety of clinical and classroom courses at Seattle hospitals and held a faculty role at the University of California, San Francisco School of Nursing. She plans to pursue a doctorate in nursing with a focus on education.

Reviewers

Erin Beauchemin, RN, CCRN

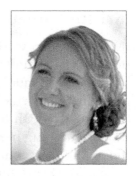

Erin is a critical care trained nurse, from Seattle, WA. She is currently pursuing her BSN, with plans to join clinical education as her career progresses. Erin is not only a team member of all technologies relating to critical care (IABP, PAC, ECMO/ELCS, Impella, CRRT, etc.), but also is a nurse advocate for research at the bedside for the nurse clinician. With a strong emphasis on cardiac medicine, she enjoys "just in time" teaching regarding hemodynamics and critical patient care management while on shift.

Natalie Alotis Lovely, BSN, RN, CCRN, PCCN

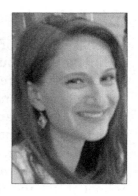

Natalie received her Bachelors of Science in Nursing from Washington State University and a Bachelor of Arts in Communication from the University of Washington. She works at Harborview Medical Center in Seattle, Washington, spending the last 4 years in the Medical Cardiac Intensive Care Unit.

About the PCCN® Exam

The PCCN® is administered by the American Association of Critical Care Nurses (AACN). Website: www.aacn.org

Qualifications to sit the exam:

► Hold a current unencumbered nursing license

► Practice 1,750 hours in the previous 2 years

► 875 hours in the most recent year preceding application

► RNs or APRNs practicing for > 5 years with at least 2,000 practice hours, only need to work 144 hours in the most recent year

► If you have any questions about eligibility, please contact AACN—they are super helpful!

The application consists of 3 pages total. Two pages ask about demographic data, one page is an honor statement. You will need to provide the name & contact information of a colleague or manager who can verify your eligibility.

Once AACN receives your application, they usually take about 2–4 weeks to process everything. Once it has been processed & you are deemed eligible, you will receive an email and postcard from a company called AMP. They will give you directions to schedule your exam. You have 90 days to schedule. Easy peasy!

The PCCN® exam consists of 125 questions. Twenty five questions will not count toward your final score. They are used for statistical data for future exams. It's kind of a bummer that you don't know which ones don't count! The advice I always give nurses—if you come across a question that you have NO idea the answer, tell yourself it's a question that doesn't count! Don't psych yourself out if you don't know the answer. There will be some questions you just don't know.

Exam questions are written at the application & analysis levels based on Synergy model of care; meaning they aren't super basic questions! They want to know you know how to take care of patients and what to anticipate in treatment! On that same thought, they also aren't trying to trick you. Each question will have 4 answer choices and only one is the correct answer!

You will have 2½ hours to complete the exam. The passing "cut score" is 68. You have to get 68 correct out of 100. Translated—you have to get about 68% correct to pass. That's it! You can easily do this! BUT, you have to go in prepared! In general, the reported pass rate for the PCCN® exam is about 75%. You can do this! (PS. The way they score is a little more complicated than a straight 68%, but I'm not completely sure exactly how that's done!)

HERE'S THE PCCN® BLUEPRINT
NEW PLAN AS OF OCTOBER 15, 2015

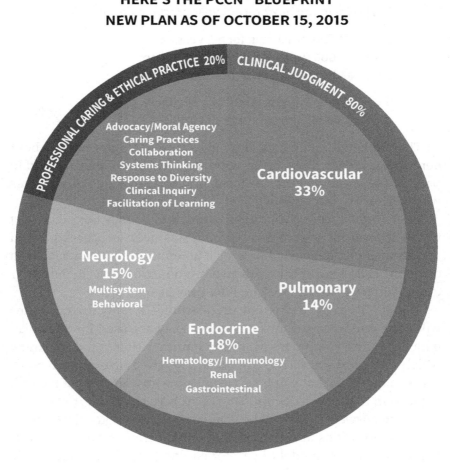

GENERAL TEST TIPS:

✓ Go in with attitude! Confident attitude!
  You can do this!

✓ Get to the testing site on time

✓ Answer every question

✓ You can change answers, but…<u>DON'T</u>!!

✓ You'll have a clock in the lower right hand corner
  of your computer screen

✓ Pace yourself

✓ You will find out right away if you passed!

Positive Mental Attitude

Words of encouragement
from certified nurses:

"Don't be afraid to challenge yourself! If you hadn't said: "You can do this!" I wouldn't have tried!"

Karen M., Oregon

"Grab this book and grab a friend, study together to ace the PCCN!"

Guy M., Seattle, WA

"Think of the first day you took your own patient as an ICU nurse. This test won't be anywhere near as scary or hard as that was."

Shenoah C. Seattle, WA

"You've studied, you have seen this in your practice. Now apply all that knowledge and pass!"

Becky B. Seattle, WA

"I know too many great critical care nurses that let the test process intimidate them and never earned the recognition they deserved, and they regret it. Don't be one of those nurses that sets a goal every year to "pass the PCCN" and never sits the test. Make it happen! It matters."

Laure L. Lewiston, ID

"The secret to passing for me was (1) Picking a time frame where test prep could be a high priority, (2) Picking a great "study buddy" who would review content and practice test questions with me weekly and (3) Practice questions!!!"

Erika G., Virginia

"Certification is a demonstration to your commitment to your professional development and your craft."

Cris G., Bellingham, WA

"I took the test to prove to myself that I could and to show my daughters that pursuit of education is a life-long adventure!"

Kelly M. Bellevue, WA

"I wanted to be the best critical care nurse possible. CCRN (& PCCN) certification was the level of excellence."

Ruth P. Spokane, WA

"Sign up with a friend—you'll keep each other motivated and will hold each other accountable to get it done!! Sign up for a date to take it and then practice, practice, practice test questions and you'll be ready. It's the greatest feeling to be certified—shows your professionalism and affirms your knowledge in your field! You can do it!!"

Mary S. Minneapolis, MN

"Set a date and stick with it! You can do it!"

Sheri R-H Newman Lake, WA

"Get certified!!!! You will feel much more valued in your career!!!!"

Archie O. Seattle, WA

"The thing that helped the most was taking practice exams with a timer in a quiet place . . . Kind of set it up to mimic the real thing so when I sat for the exam it was already well "rehearsed"."

Jesse M. Eugene, OR

"I chose to get CCRN certified not only to improve my knowledge and expertise to help better my bedside role, but to show myself I was capable and knowledgeable! It's just as much for you as it is for your patients."

Kimberly K. Portland, OR

"My advice is that you set a date, sign up for a review course and push yourself to learn as much as possible in the critical care unit. Ask a lot of questions, help your co-workers with complex patients and make a list of anything new you encounter so every day is a learning experience. Most importantly, have pride and confidence in yourself! You got this!"

Debra Beaverton, OR

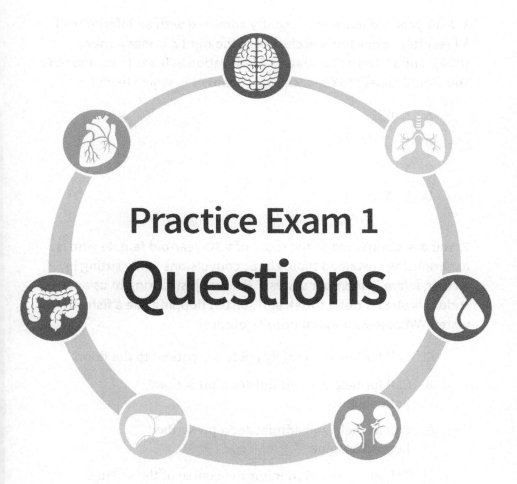

Practice Exam 1
Questions

Practice Exam #1

1. A 49-year-old male was recently admitted with an inferior wall MI resulting from 100% occlusion of the right coronary artery (RCA). The 12-Lead ECG reveals ST elevation in leads II, III, and aVF. You would expect to see reciprocal changes in which leads?

    A. I, aVR

    B. V_1, V_2

    C. V_3, V_4

    D. I, aVL

2. You are summoned to the room of a 30-year-old female who is experiencing sustained tonic-clonic convulsions while sitting in a chair. A family member states: "She was just talking to us and suddenly she let out a shriek and started flopping like a fish out of water." What is your initial priority of care?

    A. Call for help and safely guide the patient to the floor

    B. Call for help and administer a prescribed antiepileptic

    C. Call for help and administer a prescribed benzodiazepine

    D. Call for help and monitor the course of the seizure

3. A 46-year-old patient presents with pneumonia and sepsis. He was treated with 4 days of antibiotics and IV fluids. He is increasingly short of breath and is now on 100% FiO$_2$ via non-re-breather mask. You obtain an ABG with the following results: pH 7.20 / PaCO$_2$ 68/ PaO$_2$ 102/ HCO$_3$ 28. A chest x-ray reveals bilateral pulmonary infiltrates. The patient is likely developing:

    A. Worsening pneumonia

    B. Acute Respiratory Distress Syndrome

    C. Pulmonary embolus

    D. Atelectasis

4. A 56-year-old male is admitted to the PCU with a hypertensive crisis. His blood pressure is now 205/125 mm Hg and he is complaining of a headache with nausea. He reports he ran out of blood pressure medication three days ago, but also appears to be confused to the date and situation. What is the most appropriate treatment approach?

    A. Rapidly lower the systolic pressure to 100 mm Hg with IV antihypertensive medication, then gradually reduce the diastolic pressure to 85 mm Hg with oral antihypertensive medications

    B. Slowly lower the systolic pressure to 120 mm Hg with IV antihypertensive medications, then switch to oral antihypertensive medications for maintenance

    C. Rapidly lower the diastolic pressure to 100 mm Hg with IV antihypertensive medications, then continue to gradually reduce the diastolic pressure to 85 mm Hg with oral antihypertensive medications

    D. Slowly lower the diastolic pressure to 85 mm Hg with oral antihypertensive medications, then adjust dose for maintenance

5. Which of the following labs must be closely monitored when administering Lisinopril to a patient with systolic heart failure?

    A. Sodium

    B. Phosphate

    C. Magnesium

    D. Potassium

6. A 57-year-old man was admitted with an acute myocardial infarction and is rapidly deteriorating. He has a BP of 86/42 (57), heart rate of 110, weak, thready pulses, and mottled skin—especially at the knees. He has had minimal urine output the past 8 hours. A Rapid Response is activated. Which of the following medications would be the best option to increase the patient's cardiac output?

    A. Dobutamine

    B. Norepinephrine

    C. Amiodarone

    D. Phenylephrine

7. You are caring for a patient post gastric bypass. Which of the following parameters should you closely monitor after surgery?

    A. HR, RR, temperature, WBC & MAP

    B. Protein levels and vitamin B12

    C. Albumin and pre-albumin levels

    D. Signs of dumping syndrome

8. You are caring for a patient admitted after a ground level fall. The patient has decreased level of consciousness. On admission the patient is ordered to be a full code. The family arrives with advanced directives stating the patient wishes not to have CPR performed or life sustaining treatment continued. The nurse approaches the provider about this discrepancy and the provider states "I am aware of the advanced directive, but the daughter wants everything done." What is the appropriate next step by the nurse?

    A. Ask the daughter why she wants everything done

    B. Collaborate with the provider and social worker to schedule a family meeting

    C. Tell the doctor we have to follow the patient's wishes

    D. Discuss the situation with the nurse manager

9. Which is the best intervention to promote safety of the patient receiving hemodialysis?

    A. Direct visualization of the connection between the machine and the access device

    B. Strict intake and output monitoring

    C. Strict bedrest

    D. Electrolyte assessment q 4 hours

10. Four hours after starting an insulin infusion in a patient admitted with diabetic ketoacidosis, the patient's blood glucose is 235 mg/dL. Which of the following fluids should be administered at this point?

    A. Hypertonic solution to hydrate the cell

    B. $D_5.45$ or D_5NS with a glucose source

    C. Isotonic saline bolus to maintain extracellular hydration

    D. Hypotonic saline to provide cellular hydration

11. A 45-year-old male is admitted to the PCU with severe sepsis. You are administering lactated ringers 500 ml IV boluses. A central line has been placed. Which of the findings below indicate the fluid boluses are having its intended effect?

    A. MAP of 55 mm Hg

    B. $ScvO_2$ of 52%

    C. Initial lactate level 4.2 mmol/L, now 1.8 mmol/L

    D. Urine output of 15 ml/hour

12. A 72-year-old male patient has been in the PCU for 6 days for treatment of a COPD exacerbation. He has been receiving VTE prophylaxis with subcutaneous Heparin since admission. Today, his platelet count decreased significantly to 43,000 and he was found to have a new DVT on his right upper extremity. What do you suspect is the most likely cause of these new findings?

    A. DIC

    B. ITP

    C. HIT

    D. TRALI

13. Which set of hemodynamic parameters is associated with right-sided heart failure?

    A. Increased cardiac output, increased preload, increased afterload

    B. Increased cardiac output, decreased preload, decreased afterload

    C. Decreased cardiac output, increased preload, increased afterload

    D. Decreased cardiac output, decreased preload, decreased afterload

14. You would expect which of the following laboratory findings in a patient with Diabetes Insipidus?

    A. Increased serum osmolality, decreased serum sodium, increased urine osmolality

    B. Increased serum osmolality, decreased urine osmolality, increased serum sodium

    C. Decreased serum osmolality, increased serum sodium, decreased urine osmolality

    D. Decreased serum osmolality, decreased serum sodium, decreased urine osmolality

15. A 32-year-old male was admitted to the PCU with hypovolemia after a motorcycle accident. He sustained multiple injuries including a fractured tibia/fibula and a splenic laceration. Which of the following hemodynamic profiles would be consistent with a diagnosis of early compensated hypovolemic shock?

    A. Normal cardiac output & stroke volume, increased afterload, MAP 65 mm Hg

    B. Elevated cardiac output & stroke volume, low afterload, MAP 70 mm Hg

    C. Low cardiac output & stroke volume, high afterload, MAP 50 mm Hg

    D. Normal cardiac output & stroke volume, normal afterload, MAP 70 mm Hg

16. Your patient is admitted with an acute asthma exacerbation. An ABG is obtained because they continue to use accessory muscles with a RR of 38 per minute. The ABG results: pH 7.35 PaCO$_2$ 42, PaO$_2$ 82, HCO$_3$ 22. You suspect which of the following?

    A. No airflow obstruction

    B. Improvement in their condition

    C. Severe airflow obstruction

    D. Pneumonia

17. Which laboratory findings would you expect to observe in a patient with post-renal failure due to obstruction?

    A. Urine output < 100 ml/day; urine sodium 45 mEq/L; BUN: Creatinine ratio 10:1; urine specific gravity 1.010

    B. Urine output < 300 ml/day; urine sodium 20 mEq/L; BUN: Creatinine ratio 25:1; urine specific gravity 1.030

    C. Urine output < 200 ml/day; urine sodium 30 mEq/L; BUN: Creatinine ratio 15:1; urine specific gravity 1.010

    D. Urine output < 50 ml/day; urine sodium 8 mEq/L; BUN: Creatinine ratio 10:1; urine specific gravity 1.030

18. Several nurses on the unit are concerned with the accuracy of a new noninvasive device measuring stroke volume. The best way to initially address their concerns is to:

A. Research new devices to replace the existing equipment

B. Discuss concerns with the attending physician during rounds

C. Request an in-service from the device company

D. Take the issue to the unit nursing research council to investigate

19. A 22-year-old female complains of palpitations. You see the following rhythm at the monitor:

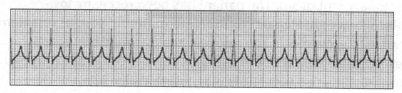

You interpret the rhythm as:

A. Atrial fibrillation

B. Atrial flutter

C. Atrial tachycardia

D. Ventricular tachycardia

20. Which laboratory values are consistent in a patient with acute pancreatitis?

A. Elevated lipase, elevated amylase, hypocalcemia & hyperglycemia

B. Elevated lipase, elevated amylase, hypercalcemia & hyperkalemia

C. Decreased lipase, elevated amylase, hypocalcemia & hyperkalemia

D. Decreased lipase, decreased amylase, hypercalcemia & hypokalemia

21. A 54-year-old male was admitted four days ago with a pulmonary embolism. The patient has been receiving low-molecular-weight Heparin for treatment. During your assessment you notice ecchymosis and necrotic areas around the injection sites. You also note that the patient's platelet count has dropped from 189,000 to 65,000. HIT is diagnosed. Which intervention should you anticipate first?

A. Stop Heparin and administer an alternate direct thrombin inhibitor

B. Administer Protamine, corticosteroids, and diphenhydramine

C. Ultrasound of extremities to assess for arterial and/or venous thrombosis

D. Stop Heparin and administer Warfarin instead

22. A 38-year-old female with a 1 week history of productive cough, progressive shortness of breath and fever is admitted with a diagnosis of pneumonia. Her vital signs are: HR 108, RR 24, BP 106/54 (62), T 38.9 ° C. What are top priorities in her care?

A. Administration of Heparin, IV fluids and SCD application

B. Administration of IV fluids, antibiotics & assessing a lactate level

C. Administration of IV fluids and Dopamine

D. Administration of IV fluids, Dobutamine and acetaminophen

23. Which acid/base disturbance is associated with massive volume resuscitation with 0.9% saline?

A. Metabolic acidosis

B. Metabolic alkalosis

C. Respiratory acidosis

D. Respiratory alkalosis

24. Which of the following medications should be avoided in a patient with a right ventricular infarction who is experiencing tachycardia and hypotension?

A. Calcium channel blockers and ACE inhibitors

B. Morphine and Nitroglycerin

C. IV fluids and aspirin

D. Plavix and Dobutamine

25. The emergency drug therapy of choice for polymorphic ventricular tachycardia is:

    A. Atropine

    B. Amiodarone

    C. Adenosine

    D. Magnesium

26. The nurse is caring for a patient admitted to the PCU after a motor vehicle collision. The patient sustained a severe cardiac contusion. Which of the following sets of hemodynamic parameters would you expect in the setting of a cardiac contusion affecting the right ventricle?

    A. Decreased cardiac output, increased right heart preload, normal left heart preload

    B. Increased cardiac output, decreased right heart preload, increased left heart preload

    C. Decreased cardiac output, decreased right heart preload, increased left heart preload

    D. Increased cardiac output, increased right heart preload, decreased left heart preload

27. A patient is admitted after being found down with an altered level of consciousness. Which of the following symptoms would indicate the patient may be experiencing alcohol withdrawal?

    A. Hypothermia

    B. Hypermagnesemia

    C. Bradycardia

    D. Tremors

28. The major risk of severe thrombocytopenia (platelet count less than 10,000/mm³) is:

    A. GI bleeding

    B. Hemothorax

    C. Intracranial hemorrhage

    D. Hematuria

29. A patient and family are struggling with a terminal diagnosis and having trouble making plans for end-of-life. The patient will be discharged home in 2 days. Consultation to which of the following services is a top priority?

    A. Chaplain services

    B. Physical therapy

    C. Nutrition services

    D. Palliative care specialist

30. Which condition is associated with an elevation in left atrial pressure?

    A. Pulmonary hypertension

    B. Tricuspid regurgitation

    C. Mitral stenosis

    D. Patent foramen ovale

31. A patient with bacterial endocarditis should be closely observed for which of the following clinical changes?

   A. Pulmonary edema

   B. Neurologic impairment

   C. Oliguria

   D. Rising liver enzymes

32. The nurse assesses a small bore feeding tube at the beginning of the shift. The feeding tube is noted to be 35 cm at the nares. In review of the chart, the feeding tube placement was documented at 75 cm at the nares after insertion. Which is the nurse's most appropriate next step?

   A. Reinsert guide wire and advance the feeding tube

   B. Instill 60 ml air and auscultate placement

   C. Hold tube feedings and obtain abdominal radiograph

   D. Remove the feeding tube and reinsert

33. The nurse is caring for a patient status post bariatric surgery on post op day 2. The patient is anticipated to discharge home on post op day 3 if the patient remains without complications. The nurse is reviewing the anticipated discharge medications which includes 50 mg extended release metoprolol (Toprol XL) daily. Which is the appropriate response of the nurse when seeing this on the discharge medication list?

   A. Review the medication with the patient and expected side effects, assessing if they have taken this before

   B. Contact the provider verifying the medication is prescribed correctly

   C. Handoff in report to the oncoming nurse to provide education at the time of discharge

   D. Discuss the medication with the patient's spouse

34. A treatment strategy for a patient with worsening pulmonary arterial hypertension (PAH) is:

    A. Imdur

    B. Beta Blockers

    C. IV Calcium Channel Blockers

    D. IV Epoprostenol (Flolan)

35. The kidneys release which glycoprotein hormone to increase RBC production in the bone marrow?

    A. Renin

    B. Aldosterone

    C. ADH

    D. Erythropoietin

36. You are caring for a patient recovering from cardiac arrest who received Targeted Temperature Management (TTM). What is the clinical rationale for providing TTM to a patient after a cardiac arrest?

    A. Prevent sepsis from aspiration during the arrest

    B. Cardiac protection

    C. Stabilize shock

    D. Neurologic protection

37. Chest pain is best described as pleuritic when it:

A. Resolves with sublingual nitroglycerin

B. Occurs only during sleep

C. Increases with deep inspiration and decreases when the patient sits up and leans forward

D. Resolves with a deep breath

38. A patient is being treated for nephrogenic diabetes insipidus with Chlorpropamide (Diabinese). The nurse should monitor closely for:

A. Hyponatremia

B. Hyperkalemia

C. Hyperglycemia

D. Hypoglycemia

39. A patient presents to your unit, post-op day 3 for a cardiac transplant. During the night the patient develops symptomatic bradycardia. Your best action to treat the bradycardia should include:

A. Administer Atropine 1 mg IV and apply 100% O_2

B. Connect epicardial pacing wires to a generator and pace the patient

C. Give Atropine and start an Isuprel infusion

D. Start a Dopamine infusion

40. Which laboratory findings would you expect in a patient with SIADH?

    A. Elevated urine osmolality; decreased serum osmolality; decreased serum sodium

    B. Decreased urine osmolality; elevated serum osmolality; elevated serum sodium

    C. Elevated urine osmolality; elevated serum osmolality; decreased serum sodium

    D. Decreased urine osmolality; decreased serum osmolality; elevated serum sodium

41. Which of the following statements is inaccurate in regard to consent for clinical care?

    A. Consent can be waived if the patient refuses to sign a consent form

    B. In the absence of an advanced directive, consent can be obtained by the next of kin

    C. Expressed consent is given directly by written or verbal words

    D. Implied consent is presumed in emergency situations

42. A patient is admitted with third degree burns over 10% of the total body surface area. On arrival to the PCU, volume fluid replacement is continued. The nurse understands volume replacement is a priority to prevent which specific type of renal failure?

    A. Intrarenal failure secondary to systemic inflammatory response

    B. Post renal failure due to calculi development

    C. Prerenal failure related to hypovolemia and decreased perfusion

    D. Intrarenal failure secondary to medication administration

43. The charge nurse responds to a Rapid Response activation for a patient admitted with abdominal pain on the medical floor. The nurse finds the patient with the following data:

BP 70/32 (44)

HR 140

RR 26

T 102.3° F (39.0° C)

SpO_2 95%

pH 7.23 / $PaCO_2$ 35 / PaO_2 88 / HCO_3 16

Lactate 4.6 mmol/L, Na^+ 140

The nurse should anticipate which of the following orders?

A. Administer 100 mEq IV sodium bicarbonate

B. Initiate Dopamine infusion at 3 mcg/kg/min

C. BiPAP 50% FiO_2 IPAP +10/EPAP +5

D. Administer 1 liter of lactated ringers bolus IV

44. Medication management in a patient post subarachnoid hemorrhage (SAH) with signs of increased intracranial pressure (ICP) includes:

A. Hypotonic saline, osmotic diuretics & loop diuretics

B. Beta blockers, hypertonic saline & calcium channel blockers

C. Osmotic diuretics, hypertonic saline & anti-hypertensives

D. Calcium channel blockers, hypotonic saline & anti-convulsants

45. A 55-year-old female presents to the ED anxious and SOB. Her 12 Lead ECG reveals a STEMI. Which of following findings suggests an absolute contraindication for thrombolytic therapy?

A. Dull chest pain, ST elevation in V_4, V_5, V_6, new left bundle branch block

B. History of cholecystectomy 2 weeks ago, ST elevation in V_3, V_4, V_5

C. Sudden onset severe chest and back pain, uncontrolled BP 195/115, ST elevation II, III, aVF, and a new diastolic murmur over the left sternal border

D. Left arm pain, BP 180/100 easily controlled on antihypertensive meds, ST elevation in V_1, V_2, V_3.

46. You are assessing a patient who was involved in a motor vehicle collision. You notice bruising around her umbilicus. Which of the following clinical manifestations would be consistent with an injury to the liver?

A. Epigastric pain, nausea and vomiting, ileus

B. Left lower quadrant pain, bloody stools, fever

C. Right upper quadrant pain, hypotension, hematuria

D. Large pulsatile mass palpated in the abdomen, lower back pain

47. Your newly admitted patient is experiencing increasing anxiety after being told she would need to stay overnight in the PCU. Which of the following interventions might help reduce the patient's anxiety?

    A. Foster dependent activities

    B. Orient the patient to the unit and discuss the plan of care

    C. Discourage problem solving

    D. Seclude the patient from external stimulus

48. The chance of regaining a pulse after ventricular fibrillation depends on:

    A. How quickly the patient was intubated

    B. The cause of the arrest

    C. How quickly the patient received defibrillation

    D. The amount of epinephrine administered

49. You are about to receive a patient with an acute GI hemorrhage. Which medication do you anticipate initiating first to help decrease blood loss?

    A. Famotidine

    B. Octreotide

    C. Protonix

    D. Sucralfate

50. A patient with pneumonia and no significant medical history was extubated 12 hours ago and is currently on 4 L O_2 via nasal cannula. The patient complains of minor dizziness and the nurse notes that the cardiac monitor is showing a regular narrow complex tachycardia in Lead II & V_1; heart rate is 182 bpm, blood pressure 94/62 (73), and SaO_2 93%. The best response is to:

A. Administer 1 mg epinephrine

B. Prepare the patient for sedation and cardioversion

C. Administer 6 mg adenosine rapidly IVP

D. Page the respiratory therapist STAT for reintubation

51. A patient who overdosed on metformin (Glucophage) was admitted to the PCU for a dextrose infusion. The RN expects the medication-induced hypoglycemia to begin resolving in:

A. 3 hours

B. 6 hours

C. 12 hours

D. 48 hours

52. During the admission process, a 25-year-old male informs the nurse that he is not able to accept a blood transfusion for matters of conscience. Which is the best immediate response?

A. "I will inform the doctor of your request?"

B. "How long have you felt this way?"

C. "I'll get the necessary declination forms for you to sign."

D. "Why don't you want blood?"

53. A patient is diagnosed with a massive saddle pulmonary embolus with right heart strain on echocardiogram. The patient requires intubation and mechanical intubation on your unit prior to transferring to the ICU. The patient's heart rate is 132 with a blood pressure of 64/32. Which intervention do you anticipate as a priority in the treatment plan?

    A. IV unfractionated Heparin

    B. IV thrombolytic infusion

    C. Subcutaneous low molecular weight Heparin

    D. Oral warfarin (Coumadin)

54. The nurse is caring for a patient recovering from septic shock. The patient has been receiving a continuous Lasix (furosemide) infusion. Which of the following interventions is a priority in the management of the fluid balance for this patient?

    A. Recording strict intake & output

    B. Estimating and documenting the patient's insensible losses

    C. Record a daily weight at the same time each day

    D. Estimate and trend a daily weight based on the intake and output from the admission weight

55. A novice nurse is unfamiliar with a device being used on his patient. The charge nurse should:

    A. Reassign the patient

    B. Help the nurse identify resources for using the device

    C. Assign the nurse a preceptor for the day

    D. Arrange for a senior nurse to assess the device

56. A patient is diagnosed with acute kidney injury (AKI) while recovering from hemorrhagic shock. The patient has been on and off norepinephrine to maintain stable hemodynamic parameters. Patient data is as follows:

BP 92/40 (57)

HR 112

Urine output < 5 ml/hour x 24 hours

Na^+ 138 mmol/L

K^+ 6.5 mEq/L

Cl 96 mEq/L

BUN 53 mg/dL

Creatinine 4.8 mg/dL

In collaborative daily rounds, the team discusses possibly transferring the patient to the ICU and starting Hemodialysis (HD) vs. Continuous Renal Replacement Therapy (CRRT). The nurse understands CRRT is the best option for this patient based on which of the following?

A. Anticipate short-term hospitalization

B. Potassium < 6.0 mEq/L & Creatinine < 5.0 mg/dl

C. Hemodynamic instability

D. Urine output > 100 ml/day

57. Signs of cardiac tamponade include:

A. Jugular venous distention, narrow pulse pressure & hypertension

B. Wide mediastinum on chest x-ray, narrow pulse pressure & hypotension

C. Widening pulse pressure, hypotension & jugular venous distention

D. A fall in systolic BP > 10 mm Hg during inspiration, absence of jugular venous distention & hypotension

58. A 65-year-old male is admitted to the PCU with syndrome of inappropriate antidiuretic hormone (SIADH) resultant from a brain tumor in his frontal lobe. The serum sodium is 115 mEq/L. What is the priority of nursing care for the patient?

    A. Fluid restriction

    B. Sodium replacement to 140 mEq/L

    C. Administration of diuretics

    D. Maintaining a safe environment

59. You are caring for a patient with a resolving myocardial infarction in right-sided heart failure that now requires preload reduction. This can be accomplished using medications that cause:

    A. Arterial dilation

    B. Venous dilation

    C. Arterial constriction

    D. Venous constrictor

60. Early signs of a proximal small bowel obstruction include:

    A. Diarrhea

    B. Fever

    C. Increased appetite

    D. Vomiting

61. Which of the following patients requires emergent pacing?

A. 2nd degree heart block Type II with 5 second pauses

B. 82 year old with complete heart block with rate of 38 & BP 108/68

C. Sinus bradycardia with 1st degree AV block

D. Junctional rhythm with a rate of 52 bpm

62. A patient s/p coronary artery bypass grafting (CABG) develops 2nd Degree Type II heart block. The patient has epicardial pacing wires. After connecting the pacing wires to a pacing generator, you notice pacing spikes indiscriminately during all phases of the cardiac cycle. Your best action would be:

A. Increase the sensitivity value (mV)

B. Decrease the sensitivity value (mV)

C. Increase the milliamps (mA)

D. Decrease the milliamps (mA)

63. A patient recently admitted with congestive heart failure is being treated with loop diuretics. What signs of hypokalemia would be evident on the ECG?

A. Tachycardia

B. Peaked T waves

C. U waves

D. Widened QRS

64. Peritoneal dialysis works on which of the following principles?

    A. Osmosis and diffusion

    B. Diffusion and convection

    C. Osmosis and convection

    D. Diffusion and diuresis

65. A patient presents with chest pain for 6 hours. Her 12-lead ECG is unchanged from 4 months ago. Which of the following would be the most appropriate for ruling out a MI?

    A. Cardiac catheterization

    B. Stress test

    C. Troponin I

    D. Transthoracic echocardiogram

66. A 52-year-old female was started on Heparin 6 hours ago for suspicion of NSTE-ACS. Her troponin is 3.8 and VSS. She suddenly complains of aching pain in her left thigh and is having trouble moving her leg. Past history reveals previous heparin therapy for suspected MI. Ultrasound reveals a large DVT of the femoral vein. Which of the following do you anticipate?

    A. Immediately stop the Heparin infusion & draw a Heparin antibody panel

    B. Prepare for administration of TPA

    C. Continue the Heparin & draw a Heparin antibody panel

    D. Prepare for stat Coumadin

67. A patient with lung cancer has the following lab values:

Serum osmo 256 mOsm/kg

Serum Na$^+$ 120 mEq/L

Urine osmo 563 mOsm/kg

Urine Na$^+$ 24 mEq/L

Initial treatment will include:

A. Desmopressin (DDAVP)

B. Carbamazepine (Tegretol)

C. Hydrochlorothiazide (Hydrodiuril)

D. Free water restriction

68. A patient who had a 3 vessel coronary artery bypass surgery 3 days ago, just transferred to your unit. Upon performing your assessment, you detect muffled heart sounds and jugular venous distention. At the bedside monitor, you notice electrical alternans—alternating heights of the R waves on the ECG. Lung sounds are clear bilaterally. What is the next appropriate action?

A. Continue monitoring as these are normal findings

B. Obtain a STAT chest CT scan

C. Notify the cardiac surgeon immediately

D. Gather supplies for chest tube placement

69. A 57-year-old male is admitted with a diagnosis of hyperosmolar hyperglycemic non-ketotic syndrome (HHNS). Which of the following should you expect as an initial treatment?

A. IV of 40 mEq potassium in 100 ml normal saline over 4 hours

B. Single IV bolus of 10 units of insulin

C. Fluid replacement with dextrose 5% in half normal saline solution

D. Fluid replacement with an isotonic solution

70. A patient is admitted with a hip fracture after a fall at home. The patient has a past medical history of end stage liver disease from idiopathic cirrhosis. Which of the following are priority principles in the management of pain and anxiety for this patient?

A. Narcotics and anxiolytics must be limited as clearance can be increased with decreased liver function

B. Narcotics and anxiolytics must be limited as clearance can be delayed with decreased liver function

C. Lactulose aids in clearance of oral opioids

D. Pain perceptions will be diminished because of impaired liver function

71. Your patient has been in the PCU for 3 days and is becoming increasingly agitated and starting to pull on IV lines. Which of the following would be the most appropriate intervention?

    A. Dim the lights and limit loud noises/conversations near the patient

    B. Ask the family members not to visit the patient because of the agitation

    C. Restrain the patient to prevent self-harm

    D. Administer sedation to decrease agitation

72. Which of the following findings is consistent with Pulsus paradoxus?

    A. Increase in SBP > 10 mm Hg during expiration

    B. Decrease in SBP > 10 mm Hg during inspiration

    C. Increase in SBP < 10 mm Hg during inspiration

    D. Decrease in SBP < 10 mm Hg during expiration

73. A 50-year-old male patient presents with acute upper GI bleeding caused by H pylori. He also states a history of coronary artery disease, Type II diabetes mellitus, and hypercholesterolemia. The provider has prescribed a vasopressin infusion to control the bleeding. What potential complications should the nurse anticipate?

    A. Hypokalemia and cerebral thrombosis

    B. Microcytic anemia and tachycardia

    C. Myocardial ischemia and hypertension

    D. Respiratory distress and hyperglycemia

74. A patient is admitted to the unit with chronic obstructive pulmonary disease complicated by acute pneumonia. The initial ABG reveals a pH 7.34, $PaCO_2$ 49, and PaO_2 63. The patient is on oxygen at 40% via aerosol mask, SaO_2 is 91%, the respiratory rate is 28 and appears mildly labored. What is the most appropriate action?

A. Titrate FiO_2 to maintain $SaO_2 > 90\%$

B. Increase O_2 to 60% and recheck the ABG in 10 minutes

C. Phone the physician to request emergent intubation

D. Set up for continuous positive airway pressure

75. You've been caring for a 43-year-old male s/p colectomy for colon cancer. You notice when his family comes to visit, he stops conversing with you and doesn't engage or look at his family. Which psychological defense mechanism is he displaying?

A. Withdrawal

B. Repression

C. Regression

D. Sublimation

76. You are caring for a patient with a chest tube drain s/p thoracic surgery. Upon assessing the system, you notice there are no fluctuations with respirations occurring in the water seal chamber. What do suspect has happened?

A. Chest tube has pulled out

B. Suction tubing is disconnected from the system

C. Air has accumulated in the pleural space

D. The chest tube is occluded or kinked

77. A patient is admitted with an acute ischemic stroke. After a head CT scan & assessment, there is high suspicion for embolic stroke. Recombinant tPA is ordered. The patient's BP is 190/125. Your initial priority is:

    A. Preparing for STAT administration of the rtPA

    B. Preparing for STAT cerebral angiogram

    C. Administer Mannitol IV to decrease cerebral edema

    D. Lowering the patient's BP to less than 185/110

78. A 56 year-old Type 1 diabetic is admitted to your unit from the OR after an appendectomy. You notice he is lethargic, difficult to arouse, diaphoretic & his heart rate is 118. Results of his capillary BG is 52 mg/dL.

Your immediate action would be:

    A. Recheck a serum glucose STAT & notify the provider

    B. Administer 4 oz. of orange juice & recheck BG in 30 min & notify the provider

    C. Notify the provider immediately

    D. Administer ½ amp of D50 & recheck BG in 30 min & notify the provider

79. A patient is admitted to the PCU with severe sepsis. The patient has a central line and you are asked to draw a "mixed venous" (ScvO$_2$) sample from the distal port. Which of the following findings is of greatest concern?

    A. ScvO$_2$ of 74%

    B. Urine output of 400 cc the past 4 hours

    C. ScvO$_2$ of 45%

    D. MAP of 66 mm Hg

80. A 62-year-old woman develops heart failure after having a STEMI. Her cardiac ECHO reveals an ejection fraction of 32%. Administering which class of drugs has been proven to decrease mortality & slow cardiac remodeling?

    A. Alpha blockers

    B. Calcium channel blockers

    C. ACE inhibitors

    D. Digoxin

81. An unresponsive 82-year old patient was admitted to the PCU after a fall at their skilled nursing facility. An emergent CT scan was performed, which revealed a large intraparenchymal hemorrhage. The patient has a known history of atrial fibrillation, for which she takes warfarin 5 mg PO daily. Her INR is currently 7.5. The nurse should anticipate initial orders for:

    A. Oral phytonadione x 3 doses

    B. Protamine 50 mg IV

    C. Vitamin K 10 mg IV slowly

    D. One unit of packed red blood cells

82. A patient arrives to the PCU for close observation, 4 hours after a high speed motor vehicle collision (MVC). The unrestrained driver struck the steering wheel on impact. Significant bruising is visible on the chest and the initial chest x-ray shows bilateral rib fractures 2–8 and a sternal fracture. The patient is on a 40% venti mask. Patient data is as follows:

BP 120/92

HR 130

RR 28

SpO$_2$ 88%

Which of the following is most likely contributing to the hypoxemia?

A. Hidden bilateral pnemothoracies

B. Aspiration pneumonia

C. Pulmonary embolism

D. Blossoming pulmonary contusions

83. A 78-year-old female has been hospitalized for 7 days with pneumonia and sepsis. She has now developed fine crackles in the bilateral lower lobes and a S3 heart sound (ventricular gallop). Patient data are as follows:

BP 90/46 (60)

HR 118

+ Jugular venous distention

The nurse reports these findings to the medical provider and anticipates which of the following orders?

A. Lactated ringers bolus 1 Liter IV

B. Norepinephrine 2 mcg/min IV continuous

C. Furosemide 40 mg IV x 1 now

D. Nitroglycerin 2 inches paste to left chest every 6 hours

84. The nurse is working with a student nurse in the care of a patient post open heart surgery. Which of the statements by the student nurse demonstrates their understanding of the risk atrial fibrillation poses to the patient?

A. "Lung collapse can occur because of a decreased pulmonary artery occlusive pressure"

B. "They can develop refractory hypoxemia secondary to a rapid ventricular rate"

C. "They may develop deep vein thrombus (DVT) due to a weak, thready pulse"

D. "There is decreased cardiac output because of the loss of the atrial kick"

85. You receive a patient from the Cath lab s/p angiogram & PCI for an acute anterior wall MI. A stent was placed to the left anterior descending artery. The patient complains of dull chest pain and dyspnea, is tachypneic, and has crackles to the bilateral lung bases. The patient has a HR of 135, BP of 88/65, cool and clammy extremities, pulses are only audible by Doppler, and no urine output since admission.

The Cardiologist has ordered the patient to be transferred to the CCU to place a pulmonary artery catheter for suspected cariogenic shock.

Which of the following hemodynamic profiles would be consistent with cardiogenic shock?

A. Low cardiac output & stroke volume, increased afterload, MAP 50 mm Hg

B. Normal cardiac output & stroke volume, decreased afterload, MAP 55 mm Hg

C. Increased cardiac output & stroke volume, increased afterload, MAP 60 mm Hg

D. Low cardiac output & stroke volume, decreased afterload, MAP 55 mm Hg

86. A 73-year-old male is admitted with a diagnosis of pneumocystis carinii pneumonia. The patient is HIV positive. On admission, he brought in a notarized advanced directive that identifies his 57-year-old partner as healthcare agent and his desire not to have his life prolonged. The patient's biological children arrive and make request to transfer their father to another facility for aggressive management. Which is the next most appropriate nursing response?

A. "I'm sorry. I'm afraid you don't have a say in the matter"

B. "Certainly. I'll get the number of the appropriate Case Manager"

C. "Let me call the doctor so you can talk with her"

D. "Have you made your concerns known to your father and his partner"

87. You are managing a patient with a traumatic brain injury and signs of increased intracranial pressure (ICP) being treated with hyperosmolar therapy. Of the following parameters, which would you expect to hold the administration of Mannitol?

A. Sodium level of less than 130

B. Serum osmolality greater than 320 mOsm/kg

C. Serum potassium < 4 mEq/L

D. Urine Output greater than 250 ml/hour

88. Priorities when caring for a patient experiencing a seizure include:

    A. Safety & DVT prophylaxis

    B. Monitoring for SIRS & preventing aspiration pneumonia

    C. Safety & administration of an anti-convulsant medication

    D. Intracranial pressure monitoring & Cerebral perfusion pressure optimization

89. A patient from the psych unit was admitted for close monitoring after drinking 8 liters of water. You would expect which of the following:

    A. Hyponatremia

    B. Hypernatremia

    C. Hypokalemia

    D. Elevated serum osmolality

90. Which of the following signs would the patient report as left shoulder pain that is indicative of ruptured spleen?

    A. Brudzinski's sign

    B. Kehr's sign

    C. Grey-Turner's sign

    D. Cullen's sign

91. An 18-year-old patient on hospital day 5 was admitted with colitis from E. coli food poisoning. Pertinent patient lab data are as follows:

WBC 23,000

HCT 20%

Hgb 6 g/dl

Platelet count 75,000

K+ 5.9 mEq/L

Creatinine 3.8 mg/dl

The provider decided to begin hemodialysis. The nurse understands the complication from the infection is:

A. Immune Thrombocytopenia Purpura (ITP)

B. Thrombotic Thrombocytopenia Purpura (TTP)

C. Heparin-Induced Thrombocytopenia (HIT)

D. Hemolytic-Uremic Syndrome (HUS)

92. Ibutilide (Corvert) 1 mg IV is ordered to be administered over 10 minutes to a patient in rapid atrial fibrillation. You know you must discontinue the Ibutilide for which of the following reasons?

A. Prolonged PR interval

B. Development of PJCs

C. Narrowing QRS

D. Prolonged QT interval

93. The nurse is caring for a patient admitted for medical management of a dissecting abdominal aortic aneurysm (AAA). The patient describes sudden onset severe abdominal and back pain. Patient data is as follows:

HR 120

BP 138/78 (98)

RR 26

O_2 94% on room air

Which of the following interventions is a priority in care for the registered nurse?

A. Administer PRN IV narcotic analgesia

B. Provide oxygen via nasal cannula

C. Administer PRN IV beta blocker

D. Complete assessment of peripheral movement and sensation

94. A patient in diabetic ketoacidosis is receiving a continuous infusion of regular insulin and 0.9% NS with 20 mEq KCL at 125 ml/hr. The serum blood glucose is now 240 mg/dL. What should the nurse anticipate next?

A. Discontinuation of the regular insulin infusion

B. Administration of a long-acting insulin

C. Change IV fluid to one containing dextrose

D. Change in frequency of blood glucose checks to every 3 hours

95. A 28-year-old male patient is day 2 status post closed head injury and T2–T5 compression fractures from a motorcycle accident. He was wearing a helmet. An indwelling urinary catheter is in place for strict I/O. Baseline vital signs: T 37.6° C, P 64, RR 18, B/P 110/60. The bedside monitor alarm summons the nurse to the room where she discovers P 50, B/P 140/68, and the patient's face is diaphoretic. What is the nurse's next appropriate action?

   A. Administer the prescribed pain medication

   B. Examine the catheter tubing for obstruction

   C. Increase the dose of sedation

   D. Perform a focused neurologic exam

96. The nurse reviews the monthly Central Line Associated Bloodstream Infection (CLABSI) report and notices that each month since the implementation of a new prevention bundle, the unit has had a CLABSI. With an interest in understanding how this is happening, which is the appropriate next step for the nurse?

   A. Email the staff on the unit reminding of the bundle practices for central line care

   B. Schedule a meeting with manager and discuss nursing practice concerns

   C. Schedule time to shadow nurses on the unit to observe central line care practices

   D. Attend unit based council meeting to hear how team members are implementing the bundle

97. A 78-year-old male is admitted with the diagnosis of non-ST elevation myocardial infarction. He is rapidly deteriorating and is placed on a Dobutamine infusion. The Rapid Response Team has been activated. His family is visibly upset. What would be your best action to assist them?

A. Teach them about cardiac risk factors

B. Counsel the family about diet changes

C. Listen to their concerns & answer questions in a way that is easy to understand

D. Discuss the cause of the myocardial infarction

98. You are preparing to discharge your patient after a diagnosis of acute myocardial infarction with asymptomatic left ventricular systolic dysfunction. He has a post MI ejection fraction of 42%. Past medical history includes MI, HTN, obstructive sleep apnea, and peripheral vascular disease. According to the ACC/AHA Guidelines for Management of Heart Failure, which of the following interventions do you expect to include in the education plan?

A. Control risk factors and avoid contributing behaviors

B. ACE inhibitors, beta-blockers, and statins

C. ACE inhibitors, beta-blockers, diuretics, and statins

D. ICD, Aldosterone antagonist, and digoxin

99. Which of the following patient characteristics accurately describes a patient's ability to quickly return to a functioning level after an insult?

    A. Predictability

    B. Vulnerability

    C. Resiliency

    D. Complexity

100. You are caring for a patient with end stage liver disease (ESLD) admitted with confusion, elevated ammonia, hypoalbuminemia, and ascites. The blood pressure has been trending downward and is now 82/46. What is the best immediate intervention to improve the blood pressure?

    A. Give a 1 liter fluid bolus over 20 min

    B. Position the patient on his left side

    C. Start a Dopamine infusion at 5 mcg/kg/min

    D. Attempt the passive leg raise technique for 3 minutes

101. A patient with severe sepsis and a new pulmonary embolism is being worked up for disseminated intravascular coagulation (DIC). Which of the following additional lab value changes should the nurse anticipate?

    A. Fibrinogen decreased, Fibrin split products elevated, platelets decreased, and D-dimer elevated

    B. Fibrinogen increased, Fibrin split products elevated, platelets elevated, D-dimer decreased

    C. Fibrinogen decreased, Fibrin split products decreased, platelets decreased, D-dimer decreased

    D. Fibrinogen decreased, Fibrin split products elevated, platelets elevated, D-dimer elevated

102. The purpose of assessing a lactate level in a patient with sepsis is:

    A. Assess for signs of internal bleeding

    B. Assess for adequate oxygen saturation

    C. Assess for signs of hypoxia

    D. Assess oxygen consumption of the tissues

103. Which of the following will cause a shift to the left on the oxyhemoglobin dissociation curve?

    A. Increased levels of 2, 3-DPG

    B. Acidosis

    C. Hyperthermia

    D. Alkalosis

104. During the admission process, you discover your patient is estranged from his family and does not have an advanced directive or durable power of attorney for health care decision making. Which of the following actions would align with being a moral agent for your patient?

    A. Tell the patient it is required by law to have a power of attorney to guide all health care decisions

    B. Put a note in the chart requesting the physician speak to him about a durable power of attorney

    C. Initiate a discussion with the patient about health care decisions and the importance of a durable power of attorney

    D. Respect the patient's wishes and do not discuss matters of death and dying during the hospitalization

105. Vasopressin is ordered for your patient who experienced a GI bleed. Which of the following patients should be monitored closely while administering Vasopressin?

    A. Coronary artery disease (CAD)

    B. COPD

    C. Liver failure

    D. Type II diabetes

106. Which hemodynamic profile is consistent with early stages of septic shock?

    A. Decreased afterload, decreased cardiac output, decreased preload

    B. Increased afterload, decreased cardiac output, decreased preload

    C. Decreased afterload, increased cardiac output, decreased preload

    D. Increased afterload, decreased cardiac output, increased preload

107. A trauma patient with multiple comorbid issues has been in the progressive care unit for several weeks and has a large surgical wound with poor healing. Which lab value is most concerning?

    A. Hematocrit 28 mL/dL

    B. Calcium 7.0 mg/dL

    C. Albumin 2.2 mg/dL

    D. Glucose 135 mg/dL

108. You are assessing a patient 24 hours after an anterior-septal wall myocardial infarction. Findings include a new, harsh holosystolic murmur and a thrill, BP 88/56 (66), HR 108, RR 35 and O_2 sat 86% on 2L NC. You should anticipate which of the following diagnostics to investigate the new murmur, hypotension, rapid breathing and desaturation?

    A. Lab work and re-administration of fibrinolytics

    B. Transesophageal echo and cardiac catheterization

    C. Intubation and mechanical ventilation

    D. Echocardiogram and cardiac surgery

109. A patient is prescribed to receive a transfusion of two units of PRBCs. The nurse verifies pre-transfusion vital signs, and consent. Patient identification and the unit of blood are also verified with another registered nurse before starting the transfusion. After fifteen minutes the vital signs are assessed and the patient is chilled, with hematuria noted in the urinary catheter. Vitals signs are as follows:

T 39.0° C

HR 135

RR 34

BP 86/42 (56)

The nurse stops the transfusion and begins infusing normal saline. The nurse anticipates the patient is experiencing what type of transfusion reaction?

    A. Delayed hemolytic reaction

    B. Febrile/non-hemolytic reaction

    C. Mild allergic reaction

    D. Acute hemolytic reaction

110. You are admitting a 56-year-old male patient with acute hypertensive crisis. As you are preparing to start IV access, you notice the patient repositioning himself frequently in bed and arching his back on occasion. What would be the next appropriate response?

    A. "Sir, please hold still while I start your IV"

    B. "How long have you had high blood pressure?"

    C. "These beds aren't comfortable at all"

    D. "I notice you are adjusting your position often. Are you in pain?"

111. A patient was transferred to the PCU after being in the ICU for 9 days. While in the ICU the patient required mechanical ventilation and was sedated on a Lorazepam infusion for the past 7 days for alcohol withdrawal. This morning's labs reveal a new anion-gap metabolic acidosis. Which of the following is most likely the cause of the metabolic acidosis?

    A. Lactic Acid

    B. Thiocyanate

    C. Ketones

    D. Propylene glycol

112. A 34-year-old patient with bacterial meningitis is admitted to your unit. The patient is extremely anxious with signs of increased intracranial pressure. The best initial intervention is to:

    A. Assess sedation and bolus as needed

    B. Open the Ventriculostomy to allow drainage

    C. Elevate the head of the bed to 45°

    D. Administer 1 g/kg of 20% Mannitol

113. A 39-year-old female is being assessed in the ED for an acute asthma exacerbation. Which of the following presentations would most likely warrant an admission to the PCU for close monitoring and treatment?

    A. Presence of inspiratory wheezes

    B. Presence of expiratory wheezes

    C. Dyspnea that interferes with activities of daily living

    D. Inability to communicate in full sentences

114. Your patient is recovering from a myocardial infarction and you now suspect he is experiencing acute mitral valve regurgitation. Which of the following findings on the echocardiogram are supportive of the diagnosis?

    A. Increase in right atrial diastolic pressure

    B. Decrease in left ventricular diastolic pressure

    C. Increase in left atrial diastolic pressure

    D. Increase in right ventricular diastolic pressure

115. A patient with severe dehydration is admitted and found to be in acute kidney injury (AKI). An arterial blood gas is performed revealing metabolic acidosis. Patient data is as follows:

pH 7.30

$PaCO_2$ 29

PaO_2 74

HCO_3 14

Which is a primary principle in management of metabolic acidosis?

    A. Sodium bicarbonate should be administered with caution to avoid overcorrection.

B. Sodium bicarbonate should be replaced until serum HCO_3 returns to baseline.

C. Respiratory compensation of the metabolic acidosis is the primary priority.

D. No fluid should be given to minimize risk for pulmonary edema.

116. You are caring for a patient requiring Hemodialysis with ultrafiltration. Which of the following accurately describes ultrafiltration?

A. Movement of water across a semipermeable membrane using a pressure gradient

B. Movement of solutes from an area of higher concentration to an area of lower concentration

C. Movement of water and solutes from an area of lower concentration to an area of higher concentration

D. Movement of solutes across a semipermeable membrane using countercurrent pressure gradient

117. As a member of the education council, you are tasked to create a teaching pamphlet for patients and families regarding their post open-heart recovery time. You plan to include illustrations and written information. What is the appropriate reading level for this type of teaching material?

A. High school graduate

B. Eighth grade

C. College graduate

D. Fourth grade

118. A cardinal sign of hyperosmolar hyperglycemic syndrome (HHS) is:

    A. Ketones present in urine & increased serum osmolality

    B. Decreased serum osmolality & rapid shallow breathing

    C. Markedly elevated serum glucose & altered mental status

    D. Volume overload & hypokalemia

119. A patient experiencing ST segment elevations in leads V_1-V_4 likely has an occlusion in which coronary artery?

    A. Left Anterior Descending Artery

    B. Right Coronary Artery

    C. Circumflex Artery

    D. Posterior Descending Artery

120. In a patient with aortic stenosis, you can expect which of the following upon exam:

    A. Narrowed pulse pressure

    B. Diastolic murmur

    C. Systolic murmur

    D. Widened pulse pressure

121. A patient who sustained blunt chest injury is admitted to your unit. The patient develops dyspnea and confusion and has distant heart tones. Two hours post admission the BP has changed from 140/78 to 92/78. The patient now has visible jugular venous distention. The most likely cause is:

    A. Hypovolemia

    B. Cardiac tamponade

    C. Cardiogenic shock

    D. Pulmonary edema

122. A 58-year-old African-American male is being discharged from the hospital status post hypertensive crisis. What is the highest priority in his discharge education?

    A. Lifestyle modification

    B. Medication side effects

    C. Signs and symptoms of stroke

    D. Smoking cessation

123. A 32 year old who experienced a traumatic pneumothorax has two chest tubes on the right side ordered for -20 cm of suction. After repositioning the patient on their right side the nurse notices a new air leak in one chest tube. Patient data is as follows:

BP 94/40 (58)

SpO_2 90%

HR 122

RR 28

What order should the nurse anticipate?

    A. 1 liter 0.9% normal saline IV bolus

    B. Fentanyl 50 mcg IV x 1 now

C. Place both chests tubes to water seal

D. Portable chest radiograph STAT

124. A 58 year old female is admitted with GI bleed. The patient has been stooling bright red blood for the past 6 hours. Patient data is as follows:

HR 114

BP 90/64 (72)

RR 22

O_2 94% 2 liters via NC

Hct 20%

Hgb 6.8

INR 1.4

$ScvO_2$ 52%

What intervention should the nurse anticipate?

A. Transfuse 2 units of PRBCs

B. Transfuse 2 units of fresh frozen plasma (FFP)

C. 1 liter normal saline bolus

D. 40% FiO_2 with CPAP + 8

125. Which of the following medications would you anticipate to administer in a patient with mental status changes due to worsening hepatic encephalopathy?

A. Neosynephrine

B. Albuterol

C. Lactulose

D. Albumin

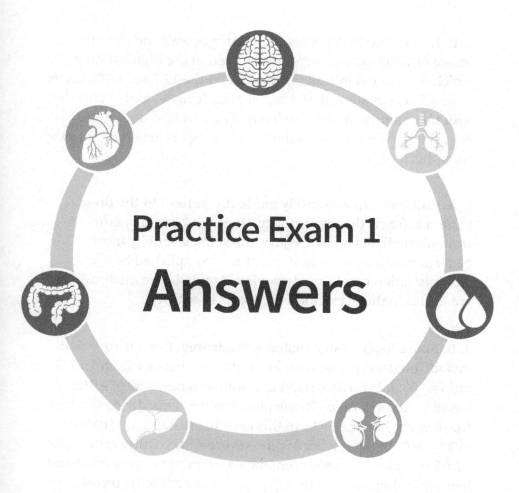

Practice Exam 1
Answers

Practice Exam #1 Answers with rationales

1. **D. I, aVL.** The RCA perfuses the inferior wall and the mirror image or reciprocal change will be seen in the high lateral wall, which is reflected in leads I, and aVL on the 12-Lead ECG. Leads V_1 and V_2 correlate with the septal area, leads V_3 and V_4 correlate with the anterior area of the heart. The aVR lead does not provide much diagnostic value as all energy is depolarizing away from this lead.

2. **A. Call for help and safely guide the patient to the floor.** Patient safety is the first priority. Once the patient is safe from immediate harm or injury, the seizure activity must be terminated. Seizure abatement is accomplished by the administration of a benzodiazepine. Antiepileptic medications are useful in the prevention of seizure of activity.

3. **B. Acute Respiratory Distress Syndrome.** Criteria for ARDS include bilateral pulmonary infiltrates on chest x-ray and a P/F ratio $\leq$ 300; it is further rated as mild-moderate-severe ARDS based on the P/F ratio. To calculate the P/F ratio, divide the PaO_2 from an ABG by the FiO_2. In this case 102 (PaO_2) $\div$ 1.0 (100% FiO_2) = 102, making it borderline severe ARDS. Other criteria for ARDS include decreased compliance, refractory hypoxemia and low expired minute volume. The patient needs to be transferred to the ICU and will likely require intubation & mechanical ventilation.

4. **C. Rapidly lower the diastolic pressure to 100 mm Hg with IV antihypertensive medications, and then continue to gradually reduce the diastolic pressure to 85 mm Hg with oral antihypertensive medications.** The patient is

experiencing a hypertensive crisis with associated hypertensive encephalopathy. This requires emergent treatment by rapidly decreasing the diastolic blood pressure to around 100 mm Hg using intravenous antihypertensive medications.

The maximum initial decrease should be no more than 25% reduction from initial presenting value. Reducing the blood pressure too quickly can lead to cerebral edema or renal failure. The initial decrease should take place over 2–6 hours. Once the BP is controlled and symptoms have resolved the patient should be transitioned to oral antihypertensive medications with a goal to reduce the diastolic pressure gradually to 85 mm Hg over the next 2–3 months.

5. **D. Potassium.** Patients taking angiotensin converting enzyme inhibitors may experience hyperkalemia. ACE inhibitors block angiotensin II, which may lead to decreased aldosterone. Aldosterone is responsible for excreting potassium from the kidneys. Therefore, ACE inhibitors can cause potassium retention and potassium levels should be monitored closely. In addition, renal labs such as BUN and creatinine should be monitored. If the patient develops more than a 20% increase in the creatinine, the medication should be discontinued.

6. **A. Dobutamine.** Dobutamine is a positive inotropic medication used to improve myocardial dysfunction on patients with a low cardiac index and elevated afterload. It will improve contractility and reduce afterload. Milrinone, which is a phosphodiesterase inhibitor could also be used as an alternative to Dobutamine, in the setting of decompensated heart failure. It is used cautiously in patients experiencing cardiogenic shock as one of the main side effects of Milrinone is hypotension. The half-life of Milrinone is about 6 hours. Norepinephrine and Phenylephrine cause vasoconstriction, which would increase the SVR and may further compromise cardiac output.

Amiodarone is an antiarrhythmic and is not indicated in this scenario.

7. A. HR, RR, temperature, WBC & MAP. Gastric bypass carries similar risks to any intestinal surgery, including the risk of an anastomotic leak. Often the first and only signs of the leak will be subtle changes in vitals or an increase in WBC. Other potential complications include bleeding, although it is rare.

8. B. Collaborate with the provider and social worker to schedule a family meeting. The patient's needs and family wishes are at odds. Communication and team collaboration is vital to patient safety and patient care that honors the patient's wishes. The nurse is a driver in advocating for collaborative communication to resolve the discrepancy in this situation.

9. A. Direct visualization of the connection between the machine and the access device. The nurse must be able to visualize the junction of the central venous access and the dialysis unit at all times. Disconnection can result in exsanguination within minutes.

10. B. D5.45 or D5NS with a glucose source. Dextrose should be included in IV fluids since the glucose has dropped below 250. This is done to prevent hypoglycemia.

11. C. Initial lactate level 4.2 mmol/L, now 1.8 mmol/L. Early goal directed therapy for sepsis includes early fluid resuscitation at 30 mL/kg to maintain the MAP greater than 65 mm Hg, $ScvO_2$ greater than 70%, and urine output greater than 0.5 mL/kg/hr. The goal is always to normalize the lactate level. The lactate clearance (lactate decreasing to 1.8 mmol/L) is a trend in the right direction and an indirect sign of increased perfusion.

12. **C. HIT.** The hallmark sign of Heparin Induced Thrombocytopenia (HIT) is a significant decrease in platelet count over a 24-hour period (> 50%) within 5–10 days of administering Heparin. The other hallmark sign is a new development of a DVT despite being on VTE prophylaxis. DIC and ITP can decrease platelet counts but with the specific scenario of a new DVT and precipitous drop in platelets the best answer is HIT. Transfusion related acute lung injury (TRALI) is a complication from a blood transfusion reaction, which causes acute lung injury typically within 6 hours of a blood transfusion.

13. **C. Decreased cardiac output, increased preload, increased afterload.** A failing right ventricle becomes congested and cannot propel blood forward to the left side of the heart, causing an increase in right sided preload; blood backs up. Decreased preload to the left side of the heart is seen as a decreased CO/CI. A reduction in perfusion to tissue prompts a compensatory response of vasoconstriction and increase in afterload.

14. **B. Increased serum osmolality, decreased urine osmolality, increased serum sodium.** In Diabetes Insipidus there is a lack of ADH. The patient will have significant volume loss leaving an increased serum osmolality, the urine will be dilute (decreased urine osmolality) and hemoconcentration of blood resulting in increased sodium levels.

15. **A. Normal cardiac output & stroke volume, HR 135, elevated afterload, MAP 65 mm Hg.** In hypovolemic states, circulating volume is depleted therefore preload and contractility are decreased which leads to a decrease in SV and CO. To compensate, HR increases to preserve CO, MAP and cerebral perfusion.

In the setting of hypovolemic shock, the HR will increase and vasoconstriction will occur to maintain the CO and MAP. A high

CO and low afterload are typically seen in early septic shock. A low CO and high afterload are commonly found in cardiogenic shock.

16. **C. Severe airflow obstruction.** In a severe acute asthma exacerbation, bronchoconstriction leads to air trapping and ABGs often show a high normal pH and low $PaCO_2$. When the airflow obstruction is severe, very little air is able to move, causing the $PaCO_2$ to rise and the pH to fall. This ABG indicates the patient is likely going into respiratory failure. Although technically this ABG is normal, it is not normal given the patient is breathing at a rate of 38 per minute.

17. **C. Urine output < 200 ml/day; urine sodium 30 mEq/L; BUN: Creatinine ratio 15:1; urine specific gravity 1.010.** In post-renal failure, there is no structural damage to the kidneys. Outflow is obstructed. The BUN: Creatinine ratio is 15:1, but both the BUN & creatinine are elevated. Urine sodium is typically 1–40 mEq/L.

18. **C. Request an in-service from the device company.** The first step in this scenario is to ensure that the device is being used correctly and solicit troubleshooting help from the device clinical representative. If problems persist despite correct use, the unit council can best determine next steps such as replacing the device.

19. **C. Atrial tachycardia.** Atrial tachycardia is caused by a singular ectopic focus in the atria that paces the heart at a rate greater than 100 beats/min. Because of the fast rate, diastolic time is reduced, thus the merging of the ectopic P-wave with the preceding T-wave. If the ventricular response rate is greater than 150 beats/min, it may be called supraventricular tachycardia (SVT). Atrial fibrillation and atrial flutter have no

identifiable P-waves. The ventricular rhythm of atrial fibrillation is irregularly irregular. Ventricular tachycardia has a widened QRS complex.

20. A. Elevated lipase, elevated amylase, hypocalcemia & hyperglycemia. Hyperglycemia, amylase & lipase will be markedly elevated in pancreatitis. Hypocalcemia and hypokalemia are seen more commonly with acute pancreatitis.

21. A. Stop Heparin and administer an alternate direct thrombin inhibitor. Heparin administration can cause HIT, therefore you should anticipate stopping Heparin and starting an alternative direct thrombin inhibitor. Assessing for secondary arterial and venous thrombosis is an important follow up. Warfarin is contraindicated in HIT until platelet activation is improving and thrombin generation is controlled. There is no evidence that shows protamine, corticosteroids, and diphenhydramine are effective treatments for HIT.

22. B. Administration of IV fluids, antibiotics & assessing a lactate level. This patient meets criteria for severe sepsis due to an elevated HR and fever. Early therapy includes antibiotics and obtaining a lactate level to help guide fluid resuscitation. Vasopressors should be utilized after fluid replacement/ resuscitation has been optimized.

23. A. Metabolic acidosis. Hyperchloremic metabolic acidosis is oftentimes associated with massive volume resuscitation with sodium chloride solution. HCO_3 is lost through the renal tubules resulting in a base deficit. Chloride replaces the excreted HCO_3.

24. B. Morphine and Nitroglycerin. A patient with a right ventricular infarction presenting with tachycardia and hypotension is showing signs of decompensation and shock.

Often when the right ventricle is infarcted, the wall motion is stunned causing a reduction in forward flow of blood from the right to the left side of the heart. To improve forward flow, the treatment is IV fluid to maximize preload (think Starling's Law!). Patients with right ventricular infarctions can become preload dependent. Medications that decrease preload should be avoided. Examples include morphine, nitroglycerin, beta blockers and diuretics.

25. **D. Magnesium.** Polymorphic ventricular tachycardia, or Torsades de Pointes, is best treated with the administration of magnesium. Other emergency antiarrhythmics have little benefit in states of hypomagnesemic induced polymorphic ventricular tachycardia.

26. **A. Decreased cardiac output, increased right heart preload, decreased left heart afterload.** Myocardial contusions generally impact the atria & right ventricle because of the position of the heart in the chest. A decrease in RV contractility can lead to decreased RV ejection fraction, decreased preload to the left ventricle, and increased pulmonary vascular resistance. Because right ventricular contractility if often impaired, blood backs up to the right atrium resulting in an increased right atrial pressure or preload.

27. **D. Tremors.** Signs of alcohol withdrawal can begin within 24 hours after the last drink and may continue for 1-2 weeks. Alcohol withdrawal may produce insomnia, delirium, visual or auditory hallucinations, and seizures. Neurologic signs of twitching or tremors should be worrisome as seizure activity may ensue. Hypothermia may be expected for a patient found down for an unknown amount of time, but is not expected with alcohol withdrawal. Hypomagnesemia would be expected secondary to long-term alcohol use and its associated malnutrition. An elevated temperature, HR, and BP is expected in alcohol withdrawal, along with diaphoresis, anorexia, nausea or vomiting.

28. C. Intracranial hemorrhage. Spontaneous intracranial hemorrhages are the greatest risk and can occur with platelet levels < 10,000.

29. D. Palliative care specialist. Palliative care practitioners excel in assisting patients and family establish an end of life plan that reflects the patient's wishes and desires. They can be key clinical partners with social work, nursing, and hospice to ensure a smooth discharge process and integration of services, both in the hospital and at home. Nutrition and physical therapy may play a role in symptom management and maintenance of quality of life. Chaplain services should be offered to the family as well but do not necessarily have the clinical acumen to aid in decision making.

30. C. Mitral stenosis. Mitral stenosis causes increased left atrial pressure during atrial contraction. Pulmonary hypertension will result in elevated pulmonary artery pressures but have no impact on left atrial preload or pressure. Tricuspid regurgitation will increase atrial preload/pressure, but not left atrial preload. Patent foramen ovale will result in reduced left atrial preload/ pressure.

31. B. Neurologic impairment. One of the risks of infective endocarditis is the bacterial strand breaking in the heart and throwing bacterial emboli forward into the lungs from the right side of the heart or to the brain/body from the left side of the heart. Neurologic impairment could be a sign of embolic ischemic stroke.

32. C. Hold tube feedings and obtain abdominal radiograph. The safest priority is to hold tube feedings and evaluate the position of the feeding tube to ensure it remains in the esophagus/stomach prior to consideration of re-advancement or replacement.

33. **B. Contact the provider verifying the medication is prescribed correctly.** Post bariatric surgery extended release medications should be avoided and transitioned to standard dosing due to absorption concerns post-operatively.

34. **D. IV Epoprostenol (Flolan).** Flolan is a potent pulmonary vasodilator used to decrease pulmonary pressure in PAH. Other pulmonary vasodilators include sildenafil (Viagra) PO, Bosentan (Tracleer) PO, and Treprostinil (Remodulin) IV.

35. **D. Erythropoietin.** The kidneys release erythropoietin when decreased levels of oxygen are detected, which then stimulates RBC production in the bone marrow. The kidney also releases renin, but this is in response to low blood flow, which helps increase blood pressure to restore renal perfusion. Aldosterone is released by the adrenal glands to help regulate blood pressure by reabsorbing water and sodium. ADH is released by the pituitary gland to help the kidneys regulate the amount of water in your body.

36. **D. Neurologic protection.** Targeted temperature management is an active treatment that aims to maintain a specific body temperature for a specific duration of time to improve neurological recovery. Managing temperature to 32–36° C for 24 hours are the recommended guidelines from the AHA. This therapy is a standard of care for patients post cardiac arrest that do not have purposeful response to commands post ROSC.

37. **C. Increases with deep inspiration and decreases when the patient sits up and leans forward.** Pleuritic chest pain indicates pain that is associated with the lungs and movement of breathing. The pain will vary based on depth of inspiration and patient position.

38. **D. Hypoglycemia.** Chlorpropamide is a sulfonylurea that is used in diabetes insipidus as an antidiuretic. It is primarily a glucose-lowering agent (used in diabetes mellitus), so patients are at risk for hypoglycemia. Other electrolyte derangements such as hypernatremia may be present in DI but are not associated with this drug.

39. **B. Connect epicardial pacing wires to a generator and pace the patient.** In cardiac transplant, the heart is denervated, so it will not respond to atropine. Pacing is the best treatment for symptomatic bradycardia, which is expected to be temporary in this scenario.

40. **A. Elevated urine osmolality; decreased serum osmolality; decreased serum sodium.** Syndrome of inappropriate diuretic hormone (SIADH) causes retention of water. Hyponatremia is dilutional due to increased water retention. Urine production is minimal and concentrated & leads to an increased urine osmolality.

41. **A. Consent can be waived if the patient refuses to sign a consent form.** If the patient has decision making capacity, then they have the ethical right to refuse treatment. It is not necessary to obtain consent if a person requires lifesaving treatment, requires an additional surgery during an operation, or if a severe mental health condition diminishes capacity.

42. **C. Prerenal failure related to hypovolemia and decreased perfusion.** Management of fluid resuscitation for burn patients focuses on the prevention of renal failure related to hypovolemia and decreased perfusion. Fluid replacement is prescribed based on burn severity and urine output.

43. **D. Administer 1 liter of lactated ringers bolus IV.** The patient is in a septic shock state with a metabolic acidosis. The initial appropriate first order would be fluid resuscitation. Sodium bicarbonate is not appropriate. After 2 L fluid resuscitation, the lactate level should be reassessed. Initiating an infusion of norepinephrine would be the appropriate vasopressor if needed.

44. C. **Osmotic diuretics, hypertonic saline & anti-hypertensives.** Management of increased ICPs include measures to decrease overall blood pressure and to decrease fluid volume in the brain. However, that is a fine balance considering the perfusion pressure needs to be high enough to perfuse the brain. Osmotic diuretics and hypertonic saline use large molecules and super concentrated solutions to pull water out of brain tissue and decrease swelling.

45. **C. Sudden onset severe chest and back pain, uncontrolled BP 195/115, ST elevation II, III, aVF, and a new diastolic murmur over the left sternal border.** Aortic dissection is an absolute contraindication for thrombolytic therapy. The findings of sudden onset chest/back pain, uncontrolled BP, ST elevation in leads II, II, and aVF and a new diastolic murmur are highly suspicious for aortic dissection and should be ruled out prior to administering thrombolytics.

46. **C. Right upper quadrant pain, hypotension, hematuria.** Typical clinical manifestations seen with an injury to the liver include right upper quadrant pain, hypotension, and bleeding. Injury to the pancreas usually causes epigastric pain with nausea, vomiting, and an ileus. A large pulsatile mass in the abdomen is commonly associated with an abdominal aortic aneurysm.

47. **B. Orient the patient to the unit and discuss the plan of care.** Orienting the patient to the unit and reality of the situation will decrease situational anxiety associated with a hospital admission. Encouraging independent activities, promoting participation in problem solving, and orienting to external stimuli can all help foster a feeling of control of their environment, thus reducing the patient's anxiety. It may be helpful to offer a tour of the PCU prior to surgery.

48. **C. How quickly the patient received defibrillation.** The length of time a patient's heart is in ventricular fibrillation is correlated with their chances of return to spontaneous circulation. The sooner defibrillation occurs, the better the chance the patient will regain their pulse. Other important clinical considerations to improve shock success include minimizing the pause before and after defibrillation and compressing at least 2 inches in depth.

49. **B. Octreotide.** The immediate treatment goals for acute GI hemorrhage focus on restoring circulating volume and minimizing any further blood loss. Generally, Octreotide will be initiated on the first confirmed evidence of a GI bleed.

Octreotide decreases splanchnic blood flow, thereby decreasing further blood loss. Patients are also started on a proton pump inhibitor, like Protonix, twice a day but it is not the first line treatment for acute hemorrhage. Antacids and sucralfate should also be considered, but not as a first line agent.

50. **C. Administer 6 mg adenosine rapidly IVP.** The patient has minor symptoms with a stable blood pressure. A 12 Lead ECG would be preferred over bedside monitoring leads for rhythm interpretation. For a narrow complex, regular rhythm, adenosine will either correct a reentry tachycardia or aid in

determining the underlying rhythm. This will assist in directing further treatment with cardioversion or antiarrhythmic medications. Cardioversion is indicated when vital signs are unstable or the patient has significant symptoms or changes in level of consciousness.

51. **B. 6 hours.** The half-life of metformin in the plasma is about 6 hours. Close monitoring is required to ensure the blood glucose level does not climb too quickly while dextrose is being administered. In a patient with normally functioning kidneys, 90% of metformin is eliminated in 24 hours.

52. **B. "How long have you felt this way?"** It is important to encourage the patient to talk about his belief to ascertain what is important to him. Initiate the conversation by determining the length of his belief. If it is a recent belief, perhaps it is a fad or there is a need for additional education or clarification. If his belief is long-standing, it has a sense of permanence and importance in his life. Option A shifts the responsibility to another provider. Option C does not encourage the patient to verbalize nor does it convey the nurse's interest in him as a person. Option D is not a therapeutic communication technique. It immediately places the patient on the defensive.

53. **B. IV thrombolytic infusion.** A saddle embolus is life threatening and requires immediate intervention with an IV thrombolytic for clot lysis. Subcutaneous and IV heparin inhibit thrombus growth and promote resolution of the formed clot, but do not produce the immediate effect necessary to treat a saddle pulmonary embolus. Oral warfarin will be started after the acute occlusion is resolved as prevention of further thrombus formation.

54. **C. Record a daily weight at the same time each day.** Daily weights are the most accurate reflection of daily fluid balance. Recording a daily weight at the same time each day is the standard to ensure appropriate fluid balance.

55. **B. Help the nurse identify resources for using the device.** The best way to facilitate learning in an ongoing fashion is to help a novice nurse identify resources such as a senior nurse or protocol. This ensures that the nurse knows where to look for help in the future. Having another nurse assess the device with the novice nurse is also useful but does not help the nurse manage the device throughout the day.

56. **C. Hemodynamic instability.** Hemodynamic instability and requirements of Norepinephrine are the biggest drivers of decision making between HD & CRRT. All other clinical data does not impact decision making between either types of dialysis.

57. **B. Wide mediastinum on chest x-ray, narrow pulse pressure & hypotension.** In cardiac tamponade, the heart is compressed by blood or fluid in the pericardial space and unable to relax and fill during diastole. Cardiac output drops, causing hypotension, and the pulse pressure narrows because there reduced ventricular volume to eject during systole. A large accumulation of blood will show up as widened mediastinum on x-ray.

58. **D. Maintaining a safe environment.** A sign of hyponatremia is confusion. Frontal lobe tumor involvement impairs judgment. Safety of the patient is of primary importance. Although Na^+ replacement would be included in the plan of care, replacement usually stops when the Na^+ reaches 130 mEq/L to prevent over-correction of Na^+ levels.

59. **B. Venous dilation.** Dilation of venous vasculature reduces filling pressures in the failing heart. The most common preload reducing medications are diuretics. Nitroglycerin and morphine are venous dilators often used in acute congestive heart failure.

60. **D. Vomiting.** When the proximal small bowel is obstructed, intestinal contents cannot move through the GI tract. GI content backs up to the stomach and often causes vomiting.

61. **A. 2nd degree heart block Type II with 5 second pauses.** For patients with adequate ventricular rate or stable vital signs, emergent pacing is usually not indicated. In 2nd degree heart block type 2, particularly with long pauses, cardiac output & coronary perfusion are inadequate and will require emergent pacing to prevent arrest.

62. **B. Decrease the sensitivity value (mV).** Indiscriminant pacing spikes indicate that the pacer is not sensing, or seeing, all the cardiac activity present. The sensitivity should be decreased so that the pacer is better able to see or "sense" the activity occurring.

63. **C. U waves.** Hypokalemia secondary to diuresis can lead to impaired myocardial conduction and prolonged ventricular repolarization. This is evident by bradycardia, flattening T waves, and prominent u waves. Peaked T waves and a widened QRS would be secondary to hyperkalemia.

64. **A. Osmosis and diffusion.** Peritoneal dialysis works on the principles of both diffusion and osmosis. Diffusion is the passive movement of solutes through a semipermeable membrane from an area of higher concentration to one of lower concentration. Osmosis is the passive movement of solvent through a semipermeable membrane from an area of lower concentration to one of higher concentration.

65. C. Troponin I. Especially in the absence of ECG changes, cardiac biomarkers are the most sensitive indicator for myocardial ischemia and infarct and will help differentiate non-ST elevation MI from unstable angina or other coronary syndromes. Other diagnostic studies may be needed to help determine location or effect of infarct, or to intervene when vessels are occluded.

66. A. Immediately stop the heparin infusion & draw a Heparin antibody panel. There are 2 types of heparin induced thrombocytopenia: one is a mild and temporary drop in platelets several days after exposure, and the other can cause life-threatening thrombosis, particularly with repeated exposure to heparin. If the latter is suspected due to clots, the patient should receive no further heparin for any purpose. A heparin antibody panel can confirm the source of this patient's clot.

67. D. Free water restriction. Syndrome of inappropriate antidiuretic hormone (SIADH) involves excess secretion or activation of ADH, causing water retention, dilutional hyponatremia, and water intoxication. Treatments are focused on promoting excretion of water and correcting hyponatremia. DDAVP and Tegretol are used in diabetes insipidus to replace or enhance ADH. Loop diuretics such as furosemide (Lasix) may be used in SIADH, but fluid restriction is the first intervention.

68. C. Notify the cardiac surgeon immediately. The signs and symptoms listed are associated with cardiac tamponade. The cardiac surgeon needs to know immediately to perform pericardiocentesis or take the patient back to the operating room for pericardial window. Cardiac tamponade is an emergent condition; if time allows, obtain a chest x-ray. Lung sounds are audible in both lung fields which rules out tension pneumothorax.

69. **D. Fluid replacement with an isotonic solution.** HHNS leads to large fluid deficits and may require multiple liters of fluid, which is determined by the patient's level of dehydration and hyperosmolality. Initial fluid resuscitation should be with an isotonic solution. Hydration & insulin will cause the serum potassium level to fall, by driving the potassium back into the cellular space. However, potassium should not be ordered as a standard dose, but should be based on the serum level and urine output.

Insulin administration should be targeted to decrease the glucose level by no more than 15% per hour. This will require a regular insulin bolus and will need to be followed by a continuous insulin infusion. Initial fluid resuscitation should not include dextrose as the patient is already hyperglycemic.

70. **B. Narcotics and anxiolytics must be limited as clearance can be delayed with decreased liver function.** Clearance of medications is delayed for patients with ESLD who have impaired liver function. Lactulose is necessary to decrease accumulation of ammonia in the GI tract, though isn't directly related to pain and anxiety management.

71. **A. Dim the lights and limit loud noises/conversations near the patient.** The initial intervention should be to decrease environmental stimulation, as sensory overload is a known cause of agitation. Dimming lights and reducing noise is helpful to decrease agitation. Asking family members to stay at the bedside may actually help reduce agitation. Restraining a patient may be necessary, but should not be the initial intervention. Sedation may also be effective at reducing agitation, but has been found to increase hospital length of stay, which can contribute to worsening agitation/delirium.

72. **B. Decrease in SBP > 10 mm Hg during inspiration.** Intra-thoracic pressures can cause compression of the great vessels during inspiration. In the setting of inadequate preload, the great vessels collapse slightly under an increase in pressure. This results in a decrease in SV that is reflected with a decrease in SBP during inspiration. This finding is suggestive your patient may be preload responsive.

73. **C. Myocardial ischemia and hypertension.** Vasopressin is given in the setting of GI bleeding to vasoconstrict bleeding vessels to promote hemostasis. Vasoconstriction also occurs systemically including coronary vasculature. In the patient with coronary artery disease, hypertension increases myocardial oxygen demand. Vasoconstriction of coronary vessels reduces myocardial oxygen supply thus raising the potential of acute myocardial ischemia.

74. **A. Titrate FiO$_2$ to maintain SaO$_2$ > 90%.** The patient is mildly acidotic, but PaCO$_2$ remains < 50 and oxygenation is sufficient at this point. In a patient with COPD, the goal is to maintain a PaO$_2$ > 60 and SpO$_2$ around 90%.

75. **A. Withdrawal.** Withdrawal is a psychological defense mechanism that patients use to separate themselves from others to avoid emotional responsiveness. Repression is when a patient unconsciously forgets painful thoughts. Regression is when a patient goes back to an earlier level of emotional development. Sublimation is when a patient diverts their energy derived from unacceptable impulses to a more acceptable social or moral use.

76. **D. The chest tube is occluded or kinked.** A small ball should tidal with respirations in the water seal chamber. If this suddenly ceases, a blood clot may be blocking the tip of the chest tube or the chest tube may be kinked so that air is unable to pass through the catheter. If the suction were disconnected

there would be a loss of bubbling in the suction chamber. If air accumulated in the chest you would notice bubbling in the water seal chamber.

77. **D. Lowering the patient's BP to less than 185/110.** Before administering this potent clot-busting agent, a patient's BP must be controlled. An elevated BP prior to rtPA increases the risks of hemorrhage.

78. **D. Administer ½ amp of D50 & recheck BG in 30 minutes & notify the provider.** The patient has a documented low glucose and is symptomatic with neurologic changes. D50 is the best option because it can be given IV in light of the patient being difficult to arouse.

79. **C. ScvO$_2$ of 45%.** A ScvO$_2$ value of 45% is of greatest concern, as it implies that the patient's oxygen demand is exceeding the supply. A ScvO$_2$ of 70% is the treatment goal and indicates a balance between oxygen supply and demand. A MAP of 65 mm Hg or greater is an additional treatment goal in septic shock.

80. **C. ACE inhibitors.** ACE inhibitors, such as Captopril, Enalapril, or Lisinopril prevent the conversion of angiotensin I to angiotensin II, resulting in lower aldosterone secretion. This results in an increase in the excretion of water and sodium thereby decreasing circulating volume, intra-cardiac pressures and venous pressures. In general, ACE inhibitors are used post myocardial infarction when the ejection fraction is less than 40%.

There is significant evidence that it decreases mortality rates of hemodynamically stable patients with left-ventricle systolic dysfunction and heart failure secondary to a STEMI. Alpha-blockers are often used to treat hypertension as they cause blood vessels to dilate which leads to a decrease in blood pressure. Calcium channel blockers are contraindicated in heart failure with a reduced EF. Digoxin may reduce symptoms but has no impact on mortality.

81. **C. Vitamin K 10 mg IV slowly.** Warfarin inhibits the activation of the vitamin K-dependent clotting factors. Intracranial hemorrhage (ICH) is considered an emergency requiring immediate reversal of anticoagulation. The recommendation for a supra therapeutic INR with acute bleeding includes the administration of Vitamin K 10 mg IV.

Fresh-frozen plasma or activated prothrombin complex concentrates, rather than packed red blood cells, would also be effective to quickly reverse the anticoagulation effects of warfarin. Oral phytonadione is recommended for an INR > 10 with no evidence of acute bleeding. Protamine is used to reverse Heparin in the setting of an elevated aPTT.

82. **D. Blossoming pulmonary contusions.** Blossoming pulmonary contusions are not detected immediately on x-ray after an injury and can contribute to rapid development of ARDS in trauma patients.

83. **C. Furosemide 40 mg IV x 1 now.** Crackles in bilateral lower lobes and a S3 heart sounds are indicative of fluid overload. Despite the tachycardia and hypotension, a diuretic is indicated. The effectiveness of the heart as a muscle is diminished in this fluid overloaded state, leading to hypotension and tachycardia. A nitrate such as Nitroglycerin, administered IV not transdermal, would decrease preload though not contribute to diuresis and a decreased fluid volume status.

84. **D. "There is decreased cardiac output because of the loss of the atrial kick."** Atrial fibrillation signature is the loss of an

atrial contraction. Without atrial contraction; ventricular filling is decreased contributing to a decreased cardiac output.

85. **A. Low cardiac output & stroke volume, increased afterload, MAP 50 mm Hg.** Cardiogenic shock results from the inability of the heart to pump an adequate amount of blood. Ischemia due to decreased coronary perfusion leads to muscle hypoxia which compromises contractility. This leads to a drop in CO and arterial blood pressure. The sympathetic nervous system responds to the decreased CO and BP by increasing vasoconstriction and the hormonal system causes salt and water retention.

In this scenario the patient is displaying signs of left sided heart failure resulting in reduced forward flow to the systemic circulation and a backup up of flow into the pulmonary system. In response to the reduced forward flow the body will compensate with tachycardia and vasoconstriction to attempt to maintain CO and MAP. The hemodynamic parameters that are consistent with cardiogenic shock would be a low CO, low stroke volume (SV), increased afterload & increased preload. The narrow pulse pressure (systole minus diastole) is also a hallmark sign of cardiogenic shock.

86. **D. "Have you made your concerns known to your father and his partner?"** This statement identifies the decision makers in the scenario as specified by the legal document of the advanced directive. The nurse recognizes a concern exists and inquires whether they have been addressed to those who have the right to make healthcare decisions.

Answer A places the family members on the defensive and is not therapeutic. Answers B and C shift the responsibility to other providers. Answer B bypasses the hierarchy established by the advanced directive.

87. **B. Serum osmolality greater than 320 mOsm/kg.** Mannitol is commonly used as hyperosmolar therapy to decrease intracranial pressure. Monitoring serum sodium and osmolality levels is recommended during the course of therapy. The therapy should be held if serum osmolality is greater than 320 mOsm/kg. The concern for sodium with this therapy is hypernatremia not hyponatremia.

88. **C. Safety & administration of an anti-convulsant medication.** The first response to a seizure is to maintain patient safety by moving to the side position and ensuring oxygen and suction are readily available. Anti-convulsant administration should occur as soon as possible once the patient is in a safe position.

89. **A. Hyponatremia.** Free water has a hypotonic tonicity. Since the tonicity or osmolality is lower than serum osmolality, it can dilute the serum sodium and drop the serum osmolality. Ingesting large amounts of free water in a short period of time can cause life threatening hyponatremia as it can lead to cerebral edema.

90. **B. Kehr's sign.** Kehr's sign is referred pain in the tip of the left shoulder pain caused by splenic injury. Brudzinski's sign neck rigidity used to diagnoses meningitis, Grey-Turner's is flank bruising and Cullen's sign is periumbilical bruising and swelling, both indicating peritoneal bleeding.

91. **D. Hemolytic-Uremic Syndrome (HUS).** Hemolytic Uremic Syndrome is a complication from a toxin released from E.coli. HUS is marked by renal failure, thrombocytopenia, & hemolytic anemia.

92. **D. Prolonged QT interval.** Polymorphic ventricular tachycardia is a known complication of Ibutilide, so the medication should be discontinued if the QT is prolonged or lengthening. Other complications include bradycardia, tachycardia, or an increase in PVCs.

93. **A. Administer PRN IV narcotic analgesia.** Blood pressure management is a priority in the care of a patient with a dissecting AAA. The management of pain is a primary driver of hypertension and tachycardia. If alleviation of pain does not minimize blood pressure then administration of anti-hypertensives is an appropriate next intervention.

94. **C. Change IV fluid to one containing dextrose.** To prevent hypoglycemia, it is recommended to change IV fluids to one containing dextrose when the serum glucose is 250 mg/dL. Discontinuation of the insulin drip will result in rebound hyperglycemia. As long as the patient is on continuous infusion of regular insulin, blood glucose checks every 1 to 2 hours is recommended. Transitioning to subcutaneous insulin is a goal, but prevention of hypoglycemia is a higher priority.

95. **B. Examine the catheter tubing for obstruction.** The patient is experiencing autonomic hyperreflexia. The disorder is seen with spinal injuries occurring above the level of T6. Among the possible causes of autonomic hyperreflexia are the following: bladder obstruction, constipation, pressure ulcers, and pain. Usually, when the noxious stimulus is identified and removed, the symptoms resolve. Checking the urinary catheter for obstruction is the most appropriate next action.

96. **D. Attend unit based council meeting to hear how team members are implementing the bundle.** The important first steps are to gather information and understand how

individuals are implementing the bundle and possible barriers to implementation. Shadowing can cause changes in behavior and emailing staff and educating needs to be followed up with feedback and evaluation of the education.

97. **C. Listen to their concerns & answer questions in a way that is easy to understand.** During an emotional response to a loved ones' illness, people need to be heard, to have their concerns and feelings validated, and to receive information in a simple manner that they can take in and process. Over time, they may have more complex questions and be open to teaching, but the immediate need is for them to be heard and updated.

98. **B. ACE inhibitors, beta-blockers, and statins.** The ACC/AHA recommendations for patients with asymptomatic LV systolic dysfunction (Stage B) include an ACE inhibitor (or ARB) and beta-blocker for all patients with a history of MI and for all patients with a reduced ejection fraction (EF).

An ICD is recommended for patients with ischemic cardiomyopathy who are at least 40 days post-MI and have an EF < 30%. Controlling risk factors and avoiding contributing behaviors is a necessary discussion point, but that is for patients at risk for developing heart failure (Stage A), not for treating a patient with heart failure.

Diuretics are recommended for treatment of symptomatic HF with reduced EF (Stage C). Aldosterone antagonists are used for patients following an MI who have and EF < 40% with symptoms of HF (Stage C) or diabetes and can be monitored for renal function and potassium levels frequently. Digoxin is the only oral inotrope. It has no effect on mortality, but may help with symptom reduction.

99. **C. Resiliency.** Resiliency is defined as the ability to quickly return to a restorative level of functioning using effective coping mechanisms after an insult or stressor. Predictability allows one to expect a certain course of events or illness. Vulnerability is a patient's susceptibility to stressors that may adversely affect patient outcomes. Complexity is the patient's ability to handle multiple systems, such as family and therapy, at the same time.

100. **B. Position the patient on his left side.** Patients with profound ascites may have so much fluid that the inferior vena cava can be compressed. The decreased preload leads to hypotension. Placing the patient on his left side can displace the fluid enough to allow blood to flow normally through the vena cava and restore preload and cardiac output.

101. **A. Fibrinogen decreased, Fibrin split products elevated, platelets decreased, and D-dimer elevated.** In the setting of DIC, fibrinogen levels decrease by at least 50% or are less than 200 mg/dL. Fibrin split products (measuring the results of fibrin degradation) will be elevated (> 40 mg/dL), platelets are significantly decreased and D-dimer will be increased in the setting of clot formation.

102. **D. Assess oxygen consumption of the tissues.** Lactic acid builds up when the body is in a state of anaerobic metabolism. Failure to adequately perfuse organs due to hypovolemia causes decreased oxygen delivery causing the lactate level to increase.

103. **D. Alkalosis.** Alkalosis causes a stronger affinity between hemoglobin and oxygen. Patients will demonstrate a higher SaO_2 despite a lower than normal PaO_2. Thus, shifting the oxyhemoglobin dissociation curve to the left. The other options cause a shift in the curve to the right.

104. C. Initiate a discussion with the patient about health care decisions and the importance of a durable power of attorney. The nurse should initiate the discussion surrounding the importance and purpose of a durable power of attorney (POA). It is not required by law to have a durable POA, but state laws do require health care individuals to provide written information about their patient's rights to make treatment decisions and execute advance directives, so one must at least have the conversation. The conversation can be initiated by any health care provider it does not have to a physician or provider.

105. A. Coronary artery disease (CAD). Vasopressin causes arterial constriction, which is useful to help decrease bleeding in the GI system. The arterial constriction can also increase afterload and decrease coronary perfusion, so patients with CAD should be carefully monitored for signs of myocardial ischemia while receiving vasopressin.

106. C. Decreased afterload, increased cardiac output, decreased preload. Endotoxins released from colonized microorganisms produce a global vasodilatation. Systemic vascular resistance is decreased leaving a functioning left ventricle unopposed. The left ventricle is hyperdynamic as evidenced by an increased cardiac output/index. Because of the increased venous capacitance, there is decreased blood returning to the heart. Therefore, preload is reduced.

107. C. Albumin 2.2 mg/dL. Decreased albumin is an indicator of protein deficiency and poor nutrition, which are major contributors to poor wound healing. The other lab derangements are not direct indicators of nutrition.

108. **D. Echocardiogram and cardiac surgery.** The patient is showing signs of ventricular septal rupture, a rare complication of myocardial infarction. The infarcted myocardial septum can rupture and rapidly cause pump failure, hypotension and shock. This patient is showing classic signs of decompensation along with the murmur and thrill. A 12-lead ECG may show AV nodal conduction delay. Early surgical intervention is the best treatment for this patient. An echo will confirm the exam findings, and may occur emergently at the bedside or in the OR as the patient is prepped for surgery.

109. **D. Acute hemolytic reaction.** Acute hemolytic reaction can occur within 15 minutes of initiation of a transfusion and is different from a non-hemolytic reaction with the appearance of blood in in urine or acute bleeding. The nurse should immediately discontinue the transfusion and notify the provider. Close monitoring of the patient should continue until the patient stabilizes.

110. **D. "I notice you are adjusting your position often. Are you in pain?"** Stating observations is a therapeutic communication technique to encourage the patient to verbalize. Certain cultures do not readily express pain or discomfort. Keen observation skills on behalf of the nurse will identify nonverbal communication and investigate further.

111. **D. Propylene glycol.** A continuous infusion of Lorazepam for greater than 3 days can lead to an accumulation of propylene glycol. Common symptoms of toxicity include anion-gap metabolic acidosis and increasing osmolar gap. Other symptoms may include renal dysfunction, hemolysis, cardiac arrhythmias and CNS depression.

112. C. Elevate the head of the bed to 45°. Among other things, an increase in ICP can be caused by venous outflow obstruction. Repositioning the patient and elevating the head of the bed should be the first intervention to ensure proper alignment. If the patient continues with signs of increased ICP or is increasingly sedate, mannitol may be indicated. Opening the Ventriculostomy to drain requires specific orders.

113. D. Inability to communicate in full sentences. The severity of asthma is determined by the degree of dyspnea. A patient with complaints of dyspnea with daily activities is considered moderate severity and will usually be treated in the ED and sent home. A patient with such severe dyspnea that results in the inability to speak in full sentences is considered life threatening. This warrants an PCU admission for close monitoring and emergency treatment.

Wheezing may or may not be present and does not determine the severity. Absence of wheezes, in a known asthmatic, is an ominous sign and is also considered life threatening.

114. C. Increase in left atrial diastolic pressure. With acute mitral valve regurgitation, a sudden increase in left atrial diastolic pressure will result because of blood regurgitating back into the right atrium. The left atrium is unable to compensate for the acute change in pressure and cardiac output drops substantially as a result.

115. A. Sodium bicarbonate should be administered with caution to avoid overcorrection. Serum HCO_3 levels below 15 can be replaced with sodium bicarbonate but should be done so with caution to minimize the risk of overcorrection and pulmonary edema. Limit the replacement of sodium bicarbonate to half the base deficit.

116. **A. Movement of water across a semipermeable membrane using a pressure gradient.** Ultrafiltration is a process utilized to manage volume overload in patients with acute renal failure. In ultrafiltration, water moves across a semipermeable membrane driven by a pressure gradient.

Diffusion is the process of the movement of solutes from an area of higher concentration to an area of lower concentration. Convection is the process of combining ultrafiltration with a countercurrent pressure gradient to drag small and large solutes across a semipermeable membrane.

117. **D. Fourth grade.** While the majority of patients are literate at the eighth grade reading level, a significant amount read at or below the fifth grade level. Hence, any patient teaching materials should be written at the fourth grade level and include simple illustrations.

118. **C. Markedly elevated serum glucose & altered mental status.** Patients presenting with HHS have markedly elevated glucose levels, often greater than 1000 mg/dL. They also present with confusion or altered mental status, hypovolemia, and elevated sodium levels. Other electrolytes such as potassium, magnesium and phosphate are usually deficient. Rapid shallow breathing and the presence of ketones are consistent with DKA.

119. **A. Left Anterior Descending Artery.** The LAD perfuses the septum and left anterior wall, which are reflected in chest leads V_1-V_4. The RCA perfuses the inferior wall, right ventricle and right atrium. In 90% of the population, the RCA also perfuses the posterior wall, in 10% the left circumflex perfuses it. The left circumflex also perfuses the left lateral wall of the left ventricle.

120. **C. Systolic murmur.** The aortic valve is open during systole to allow blood to be ejected from the LV into the aorta. When the aortic valve is stenosed and stiff, it cannot fully open, so a systolic murmur is heard as blood is pushed through the narrow valve.

121. **B. Cardiac tamponade.** Blunt injury to the cardiac muscle can cause bruising, swelling, and bleeding into the pericardial sac, all of which inhibit normal cardiac wall motion. With limited stretch, cardiac output falls and blood backs up into the jugular veins, causing hypotension and JVD. Heart tones are muffled due to the fluid/blood surrounding the heart limiting movement.

122. **C. Signs and symptoms of stroke.** The patient has non-modifiable risk factors for stroke (sex, race, and history of hypertension). Priority is given to education on early recognition of stroke and activation of EMS should the signs occur. Early stroke identification and early access to a stroke center will provide the best outcome.

123. **D. Portable chest radiograph STAT.** The nurse should anticipate a chest x-ray order first to evaluate the possibility of re-accumulation of Pnemothoracies or changes in the pleural space with movement and repositioning. The chest tubes should not be put to water seal with the development of a new air leak.

124. **A. Transfuse 2 units of PRBCs.** In general, the goal for $ScvO_2$ is > 70% in the care of a patient bleeding demonstrating a SIRS response. It is important to meet oxygen tissue demands. Since the patient is bleeding, the focus needs to be on increasing oxygen delivery. Increasing the FiO_2 does not impact oxygen delivery. Since the patient has lost a significant amount of

blood, it is appropriate to treat with a blood transfusion versus a normal saline bolus. This is indicated to increase oxygen delivery to offset an increased extraction ratio.

125. **C. Lactulose.** Lactulose is a laxative that promotes frequent bowel movements as well as pulling ammonia from the bloodstream into the gut for excretion. Since hepatic encephalopathy results from decreased hepatic filtering resulting in elevated ammonia levels, lactulose is a first line therapy for patients.

You can do it!

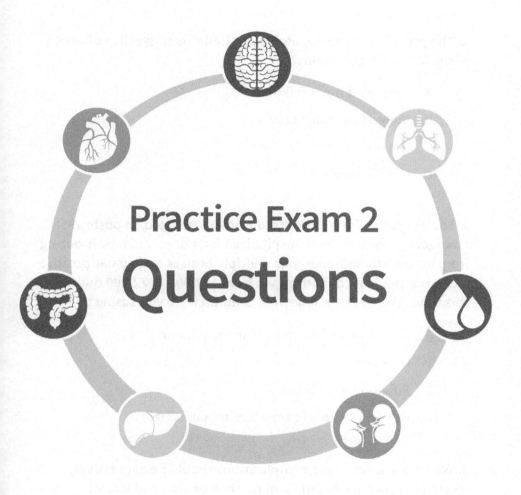

Practice Exam 2
Questions

Practice Exam #2

1. The presence of the Hepatojugular Reflex is suggestive of which of the following conditions?

    A. Left-sided heart failure

    B. Right-sided heart failure

    C. Hepatic failure

    D. Carotid stenosis

2. You are caring for a 36 year old who experienced an obstetric emergency. She has been hospitalized for 4 days and now is oozing from mucous membranes, has multiple bruises and guaiac positive stool. Her platelet count dropped from 180,000 to 22,000 during this time. Which of the following conditions do you suspect?

    A. Disseminated intravascular coagulation (DIC)

    B. GI bleed

    C. Pulmonary embolus

    D. Heparin induced thrombocytopenia (HIT)

3. Which of the following complications should be aggressively treated to prevent worsening of cerebral edema and infarct expansion after an acute ischemic stroke?

    A. Hypernatremia

    B. Fever

    C. Hypokalemia

    D. Hypoglycemia

4. A 35-year-old patient has a splenic laceration, pulmonary contusion, multiple rib fractures and a left femur fracture after a motor vehicle collision. Vital signs: HR 110, BP 94/56 (68), SpO$_2$ 93% on 40% venturi mask, RR 26, pain 4/10 with movement. What is the next intervention?

    A. Medicate for pain

    B. Teach incentive spirometer use

    C. Increase O$_2$ to 50%

    D. Bolus 500 ml isotonic fluid

5. Which of the following electrolyte imbalances can contribute to a prolonged QT interval?

    A. Hypermagnesemia

    B. Hypomagnesemia

    C. Hypernatremia

    D. Hypercalcemia

6. A patient with heart failure reports a dry, hacking cough. Her current medications include captopril (Capoten) 50 mg twice daily, furosemide (Lasix) 40 mg twice daily, spironolactone (Aldactone) 25 mg daily, and warfarin (Coumadin) 2.5 mg daily. Which change to the medication regimen should the nurse anticipate?

    A. Discontinue captopril, add losartan (Cozaar) 50 mg daily

    B. Increase furosemide to 60 mg twice daily, discontinue captopril

    C. Decrease furosemide to once daily, add losartan (Cozaar) 50 mg daily

    D. Discontinue spironolactone, decrease warfarin to 2 mg daily

7. You are caring for a 51-year-old male in DKA. To help assess the effectiveness of treatment, which of the following components are needed to determine his anion gap based on serum laboratory tests?

    A. Sodium, glucose, BUN

    B. Sodium, potassium, chloride, bicarbonate

    C. Potassium, chloride, glucose

    D. Urine and serum creatinine levels

8. Which of the following is an anticipated hemodynamic change in care of an individual with systemic inflammatory response (SIRS) in the setting of severe sepsis?

    A. Decreased cardiac output (CO)

    B. Increased pressure in the pulmonary vascular beds

    C. Increased left atrial preload

    D. Decreased right atrial preload

9. While assessing your patient, you note increasing anxiety when discussing the need to stay overnight in the hospital. Which of the following clinical manifestations would be related to the patient's anxiety?

    A. Nausea, diarrhea, shortness of breath

    B. Diarrhea, pinpoint pupils, shallow breathing

    C. Shortness of breath, sweating, dysphagia

    D. Dilated pupils, polyuria, sweating

10. Medical history of which of the following diagnosis elevates a patient's risk for developing acute kidney injury?

    A. Peripheral artery disease, COPD, myocardial infarction

    B. Diabetes, obesity, asthma

    C. Asthma, gout, hypertension

    D. Hypertension, peripheral artery disease, diabetes

11. A patient suddenly experiences ventricular fibrillation. Your immediate treatment plan would include:

    A. Chest compressions, amiodarone, & atropine

    B. Defibrillation, magnesium & chest compressions

    C. Chest compressions, airway management & epinephrine

    D. Defibrillation, chest compressions & airway management

12. The nurse is caring for a patient who is four days status post sigmoidectomy with colostomy placement. Upon assessment, the nurse finds diminished breath sounds to the bilateral lower lobes. The patient's vital signs are as follows:

BP 110/70

HR 112

RR 30

T 100.1° F (37.8° C)

SpO_2 90% on room air

Which order should the nurse anticipate?

A. STAT Chest CT Angiogram

B. Chest x-ray & pulmonary hygiene

C. 1 gram Vancomycin IV q 12 hours

D. Albuterol (Proventil) Nebulizers q 8 hours

13. A patient is admitted with acute necrotizing pancreatitis. What should the nurse anticipate as the priority step in nutrition management for this patient?

A. Begin regular diet once serum amylase and Lipase return to zero

B. Begin feedings via jejunal route to minimize pancreatic stimulation

C. Administer TPN until patient is free of abdominal pain

D. Maintain NPO status for minimum of seven days

14. A 25-year-old male patient was admitted to the PCU yesterday with a diagnosis of closed head injury. During bedside handoff, the off-going nurse reported the patient was awake, alert, and oriented to person, place, time, and situation. During visiting time, the family reports the patient "seems sleepier than yesterday". What is the appropriate next nursing action?

A. Ask the family members not to overstimulate the patient

B. Notify the physician of the neurologic change

C. Perform a focused neurologic exam

D. Reassure the family this is a normal finding in the first 24 to 48 hours

15. Which of the following medications are not routinely used for the treatment of metabolic syndrome?

    A. Oral hyperglycemic agents or subcutaneous insulin

    B. Anti-hypertensives

    C. Antibiotics

    D. Lipid lowering agents

16. You are evaluating a 12-lead ECG and notice positive deflection of the QRS complex in Lead I and negative deflection of the QRS complex in Lead aVF. What is the patient's electrical axis?

    A. Normal axis

    B. Left axis deviation

    C. Right axis deviation

    D. Extreme right axis deviation

17. A patient presents with decreased LOC and tachypnea. ABG results: pH 7.30, $PaCO_2$ 28, PaO_2 90, HCO_3 19. Ketones are present in serum & urine, serum osmolality is 320, serum sodium 132, anion gap is 20. Based on these lab findings, you suspect the following diagnosis:

    A. Hyperosmolar Hyperglycemic State (HHS)

    B. Diabetic ketoacidosis (DKA)

    C. Diabetes insipidus

    D. Adrenal crisis

18. Which electrolyte disturbance is common with patients on ACE-inhibitors, angiotensin receptor blockers, or aldosterone receptor blockers?

    A. Hypercalcemia

    B. Hypermagnesemia

    C. Hyperphosphatemia

    D. Hyperkalemia

19. A patient with ESKD presents with mental status changes after he skipped dialysis for 3 days. His ABG reveals the following: pH 7.28/ PaCO$_2$ 32/ PaO$_2$ 180/ HCO$_3$ 20. After analyzing the results, you know the patient has:

    A. Uncompensated respiratory alkalosis

    B. Partially compensated respiratory acidosis

    C. Uncompensated metabolic alkalosis

    D. Partially compensated metabolic acidosis

20. A patient with acute pancreatitis should be monitored for which of the following physical assessment findings indicating an electrolyte imbalance?

    A. Chvostek sign

    B. Kehr's sign

    C. Kernig's sign

    D. Cullen's sign

21. An 80-year-old patient is postoperative day three following an aortic valve replacement. At 17:00 the patient becomes agitated, restless, and begins pulling out tubes and devices. The provider prescribes Haldol 2 mg IV x 1. Prior to administration of the medication the nurse understands the importance of collecting which of the following patient data to ensure safety with medication administration?

    A. Completion of the Confusion Assessment Method (CAM) and 12 Lead ECG

    B. Point of care blood glucose

    C. Urinalysis

    D. 12 Lead ECG & Straight Catheterization

22. Your patient has been in surgery for 4 hours for a femoral-popliteal bypass. The husband is angry because he thought the surgery would be completed in 2 hours. What would be your best response to him?

    A. Call security in case his anger escalates

    B. Call the OR to get a status report and notify him of the reason for the delay

    C. Tell him you are unsure of the cause of the delay and ask him to return to the waiting room

    D. Call his family to be with him

23. A patient returns to your unit after implantation of a permanent dual chamber pacemaker. You note the patient is in atrial fibrillation. What would be the pacing mode indicated for this patient?

    A. DDD

    B. VVI

    C. DVI

    D. VAT

24. Which cells of the pancreas produce glucagon?

    A. Alpha cells

    B. Beta cells

    C. Delta cells

    D. Kappa cells

25. A S_4 heart sound is expected in which of the following?

    A. Pericarditis

    B. Left ventricular failure

    C. Ventricular hypertrophy

    D. Bundle branch block

26. A 56-year-old suffered a cardiopulmonary arrest & received 45 minutes of chest compressions. He has recovered, but has severe short term memory loss. On day 3 of his hospital stay, you notice his urine drainage bag is suddenly full. The urine is clear without color. He continues with UOP of 700-1000 mL per hour x 2 hours. Which of the following assessment findings would you expect?

    A. Serum sodium level of 126

    B. Serum osmolality of 320

    C. Urine specific gravity of 1.025

    D. Serum potassium of 3.5

27. A PCU patient has been hospitalized for 3 days with pneumonia. The nurse notes new facial weakness and slurred speech. Which element of the patient's medical record will be most crucial in determining treatment?

    A. History of myocardial infarction 10 years ago

    B. Allergy to contrast dye

    C. Aspirin 325 mg PO daily

    D. Gastrointestinal bleeding 2 months ago

28. You are caring for a patient who was admitted with an occluded ventricular/peritoneal shunt. Earliest signs of increased intracranial pressure (ICP) include:

    A. Nystagmus

    B. Decreased level of consciousness

    C. Slurred speech

    D. Unequal pupils

29. You administer Albuterol nebulizers to a patient having an asthmatic exacerbation. Their initial ABG was: pH 7.45/PaCO$_2$ 28/ PaO$_2$ 142/HCO$_3$ 22. An ominous sign of impending respiratory failure includes:

    A. Respiratory alkalosis

    B. Hypercapnia

    C. Hypoxemia

    D. Metabolic acidosis

30. You are caring for a patient diagnosed with nephrogenic diabetes insipidus. Which of the following correctly identifies the cause of this disorder?

    A. Insufficient insulin production

    B. Ingestion of excessive amount of water resulting in suppression of vasopressin release

    C. The kidneys are not responding appropriately to vasopressin (ADH)

    D. Deficiency of vasopressin production secondary to damage to the posterior pituitary

31. Some common clinical manifestations of cardiogenic shock would include:

    A. Decreased afterload

    B. Decreased preload

    C. Expiratory wheezes

    D. Cool, pale, moist skin

32. You are caring for a patient decompensating with a suspicion of development of septic shock. The Rapid Response Team is activated. Three liters of fluid have been administered; however the patient is still experiencing hypotension with minimal urine output. The provider has ordered vasopressor therapy. According to the Sepsis Guidelines, which of the following vasopressors is recommended for treating hypotension?

    A. Dobutamine

    B. Dopamine

    C. Norepinephrine

    D. Vasopressin

33. A new nursing staff member recently relocated to the area. After starting on their new unit, the nurse notices different practices related to the care of central lines and IV tubing from what they were trained to do from the previous organization. After reviewing established standards of care for central lines through their national nursing organization, what is the most appropriate next step by the nurse?

    A. Email the manager and tell them about the discrepancies assessed

    B. Email the staff with the information attached drawing their attention to the concerning practices

    C. Email the unit practice council chair and ask to have this added to the next meeting agenda

    D. Bring this concern to the morning huddle for discussion

34. A 45-year-old patient is scheduled to go to the cardiac catheterization lab in the morning for a coronary angiogram. Which of the following is most effective to prevent contrast induced nephropathy?

A. Acetylcysteine (Mucomyst) 1500 mg PO/NG q 12 hours x 6 doses

B. Lactated ringers at 100 ml/hour 12 hours before and after the procedure

C. Furosemide (Lasix) 20 mg IV q 6 hours x 4 doses

D. Mannitol 25% 0.5 grams/kg of body weight IV over 30 min

35. A nurse is educating the family of a patient with acute coronary syndrome about potential treatments. What is the most accurate statement?

A. "Percutaneous coronary intervention is the best therapy for MI"

B. "Fibrinolytics are preferred for non-ST elevation MI"

C. "Percutaneous coronary intervention should be completed within 4 hours of arrival"

D. "Treatment will be determined based on symptoms and lab work"

36. Which of the following should be avoided in a patient with a basilar skull fracture?

    A. Nasogastric tubes

    B. Urinary catheters

    C. Fevers

    D. Central lines

37. Pharmaceutical management of hypertrophic cardiomyopathy should include:

    A. Metoprolol (Lopressor)

    B. Furosemide (Lasix)

    C. Digoxin (Lanoxin)

    D. Nitroprusside (Nipride)

38. A patient with viral pneumonia has been hospitalized for 10 days. You noticed the serum sodium level is consistently dropping and is now 124. You request additional labs and find the serum osmo is 248, urine output has been about 600 ml/day.

These findings are consistent with:

    A. Diabetes insipidus (DI)

    B. Dilutional hyponatremia

    C. Adrenal Crisis

    D. Diabetic Ketoacidosis (DKA)

39. When administering vasoactive drugs, which of following parameters most accurately estimates end-organ perfusion?

A. Urinary output, lactate, $ScvO_2$

B. Pulse, urinary output, strength of pulses

C. Blood pressure, respiratory rate, ST depression on 12 Lead ECG

D. Urinary output, white blood cell count, temperature

40. When caring for a patient of Asian descent, it is important to assess the level of pain as well as which of the following?

A. The Faces Pain Scale

B. Cultural norms for pain expression

C. Disregard the patient's cultural factors

D. Use clinical judgment about the level of pain

41. While assessing a patient, the RN notes a systolic ejection murmur, split S2, and rales. These findings are consistent with:

A. Mitral stenosis

B. Mitral regurgitation

C. Aortic stenosis

D. Aortic regurgitation

42. You are caring for a patient with suspected thrombocytopenia. Which of the following physical assessment findings would be expected in the setting of thrombocytopenia?

    A. Petechiae

    B. Erythema

    C. Blood clots in the urinary catheter tubing

    D. Pitting edema

43. Your patient is recovering from laparoscopic gastric bypass surgery. Which of the following potential complications do you anticipate most once the patient starts eating?

    A. Dumping syndrome

    B. Acute renal failure

    C. Diabetes mellitus

    D. Pancreatitis

44. A spiral CT scan reveals a pulmonary embolism in a 38-year-old with stable vital signs. You should prepare for which of the following?

    A. Coumadin with daily PT/INR monitoring

    B. rtPA infusion—80 mg over 1 hour

    C. Unfractionated heparin with daily PTT, adding Coumadin after 1–2 days

    D. Pradaxa anticoagulation therapy

45. While precepting a new orientee you observe the orientee performing a task utilizing a different method than the way you originally demonstrated. What would be the appropriate response?

A. Tell the orientee they are doing it incorrectly and they must do it as taught

B. Perform a literature review to determine best practice

C. Survey other staff to get a feel for their methods

D. Ignore the difference and assume the orientee knows the correct method

46. You are summoned immediately to the room of a 30-year-old female who is experiencing sustained tonic-clonic convulsions while sitting in a chair. A family member states: "She was just talking to us and suddenly she let out a shriek and started flopping like a fish out of water." What is your priority of care?

A. Call for help and safely guide the patient to the floor

B. Call for help and administer a prescribed antiepileptic

C. Call for help and administer a prescribed benzodiazepine

D. Call for help and monitor the course of the seizure

47. A patient recovering from Roux-en-Y gastric bypass surgery is using her CPAP on her normal home settings. She is complaining of abdominal pain that does not seem to be related to her incisions. Vital signs show the following:

HR 125

BP 88/42 (57)

RR 30

SpO_2 92%

T 100.5° F (38.1° C)

What is the appropriate action?

    A. Initiate the sepsis protocol

    B. Administer acetaminophen (Tylenol) 650 mg PO

    C. Notify the provider of a potential anastomotic leak

    D. Notify the provider and request an increase in her CPAP settings

48. Which is the immediate stimulus that initiates the renin-angiotensin-aldosterone system?

    A. Reduced cerebral perfusion pressure

    B. Hyponatremia

    C. Reduced left ventricular end diastolic pressure

    D. Reduced renal perfusion pressure

49. You are reviewing the 12-lead ECG of a patient presenting with substernal chest pressure for 4 hours. You see ST-segment elevation in leads II, III, and aVF. You also see ST-segment depression in leads V_1 and V_2 with a large R-wave in V_2. What type of MI do you suspect?

    A. Infero-septal

    B. Infero-posterior

    C. Infero-lateral

    D. Inferior only with reciprocal changes in V_1 and V_2

50. You are performing heart tone assessment and hear a murmur loudest at the 5ᵗʰ ICS, left midclavicular line. You palpate the radial pulse and hear the murmur on the S₂ heart sound. What type of murmur do you suspect?

A. Aortic regurgitation

B. Mitral regurgitation

C. Aortic stenosis

D. Mitral stenosis

51. A patient with heparin-induced thrombocytopenia (HIT) needs to be monitored for which of the following complications?

A. Disseminated Intravascular Coagulation (DIC)

B. Hemorrhagic stroke

C. Transient Ischemic Attack (TIA)

D. Ischemic stroke

52. A patient receiving Vancomycin for a severe staphylococcus infection has a new order for Gentamicin in addition to their current regimen. Which of the following lab values does the nurse understand is necessary to review with the provider prior to administration of the antibiotic?

A. Creatinine 2.8 mg/dL

B. Serum potassium 3.4 mEq/L

C. Serum sodium 145 mmol/L

D. White Blood Cells (WBCs) 3000/mm³

53. A Rapid Response is activated on a patient post-operative day 3 from a subdural hematoma (SDH) evacuation. The patient is transferred to the ICU. Which of the following would be most concerning for a new left-sided subdural hematoma?

A. Bilateral pinpoint non-reactive pupils

B. Right pupil greater than left and minimally reactive

C. Left pupil greater than right and minimally reactive

D. Bilateral pupils 6 cm with brisk reaction

54. You are assisting with a central line placement and your patient acutely develops dyspnea, tachycardia, decreased oxygen saturation, and right-sided chest pain. The provider suspects a pneumothorax. Which of the following interventions should be implemented as a priority?

A. Administer analgesics

B. Administer antibiotics

C. Chest tube insertion

D. Echocardiogram

55. Which of the following laboratory findings would be expected in the diuretic phase of Acute Tubular Necrosis (ATN)?

A. Decreased urine osmolality

B. Decreased BUN: Creatinine ratio

C. Hypophosphatemia

D. Decreased urine sodium

56. Symptoms most commonly associated with mitral insufficiency include:

    A. Systolic murmur

    B. Pulsus paradoxus

    C. Mid-diastolic click

    D. Jugular venous distention

57. EMS arrives with a patient that was found down on the sidewalk outside of the local tavern. When assessing your patient's abdomen you notice ecchymosis in the lower abdomen and flank region. This is known as_____ and is indicative of _____?

    A. Kernig's sign; intra-abdominal bleeding

    B. Cullen's sign; meningitis

    C. Grey-Turner's sign; retroperitoneal bleed

    D. Brudzinski's sign; occlusion of the mesenteric artery

58. Mrs. Jensen is a 45-year old patient who has metastatic breast cancer and is complaining of bone pain. During the physical assessment you note crackles through the mid lung fields and bases and chest radiograph verifies pulmonary edema. In addition, the calcium level is noted at 13.1 mg/dL when reviewing her labs. Which of the following diuretics would you expect the provider to order for the patient?

    A. Mannitol

    B. Hydrochlorothiazide

    C. Spironolactone

    D. Furosemide

59. Which finding would help distinguish neurogenic from other forms of distributive shock?

    A. BP 80/45 (57)

    B. HR 45 bpm

    C. Increased afterload

    D. Normal cardiac output

60. An 18-year-old with Type 1 diabetes is admitted with a hyperglycemic emergency. Her initial glucose was 320 mg/dL with a potassium of 5.2.

Your highest priority when caring for her is:

    A. Correcting her glucose levels

    B. Ensuring she eats dinner

    C. Restarting her home SQ insulin

    D. Correcting her fluid deficit

61. Which set of potential complications are most commonly associated with acute pancreatitis?

    A. ARDS, DIC, and hypovolemic shock

    B. Stroke, pulmonary embolism, and acute MI

    C. Tension pneumothorax, cardiac tamponade, and chylothorax

    D. Acute liver failure, DIC, and acute renal failure

62. A 29-year-old male is admitted to the PCU after multiple bee stings while hiking. The patient has complaints of uticaria. Upon further assessment which of the following findings would raise the most concern?

A. Voice hoarseness

B. HR 55

C. WBC count of 14,000

D. Temperature of 38° C (100.4° F)

63. A 67-year-old patient with history of COPD and atrial fibrillation is admitted for acute respiratory failure. Medication management will include which of the following?

A. Theophylline (Theo-24)

B. Subcutaneous epinephrine (EpiPen)

C. Alprazolam (Xanax)

D. Glycopyrrolate (Robinul)

64. A patient admitted with heart failure develops hypotension, tachycardia, decreasing LOC, cool clammy skin, decreasing UOP & tachypnea. Which of the following would be included in the patient's plan of care?

A. Positive inotropic agents, diuretics & vasodilators

B. ACE Inhibitors, adenosine, beta blockers

C. Beta blockers, diuretics, calcium channel blockers

D. Negative inotropic medications, digoxin, antidysrhythmics

65. A 68-year-old patient presents to your unit 9 days after a 3 vessel CABG complaining of chest pain. A 12-lead ECG reveals non-specific ST elevation in leads V_1–V_6. Cardiac enzymes are not elevated. He states the pain is better when he sits up and leans forward. This scenario is most consistent with:

    A. Acute inferior wall MI

    B. Post-operative cardiac tamponade

    C. Pleural effusions

    D. Pericarditis

66. A major goal for a patient who is 48 hours s/p valve replacement surgery is to:

    A. Administer antibiotics

    B. Stabilize hemodynamics

    C. Prevent thrombus formation

    D. Promote diuresis

67. You are caring for a 48-year-old with gram negative rod sepsis. She has been hospitalized for 3 days and now is oozing from mucous membranes, has multiple bruises and guaiac positive stool. There is suspicion for Disseminated Intravascular Coagulation (DIC). Which of the following lab values do you suspect?

    A. Decreased platelets, increased fibrinogen, decreased D-dimer

    B. Decreased platelets, decreased fibrinogen, increased D-dimer

    C. Increased platelets, decreased fibrinogen, increased D-dimer

    D. Increased platelets, increased fibrinogen, increased D-dimer

68. A 74-year-old patient is admitted to the PCU with a diagnosis of atrial fibrillation with a rapid ventricular response and dyspnea. The patient starts to have complaints of arm weakness and you notice slurred speech. The patient is emergently taken to CT scan and is diagnosed with an ischemic stroke. Which of the following is an exclusion criterion for administering thrombolytic therapy such as rtPA?

    A. Patient is over the age of 18

    B. Less than 3 hours since the onset of stroke symptoms

    C. Seizure activity with onset of stroke symptoms

    D. Neuro deficit is detected while performing the NIH stroke scale

69. A 19-year-old female is admitted to the PCU with nausea/vomiting, and Kussmaul's respirations at a rate of 26. Serum blood glucose is 320 mg/dL. What is the priority of management?

    A. Administration of antiemetic medication

    B. Oxygen via nasal cannula at 4 L/min

    C. IV Insulin administration

    D. Volume resuscitation

70. A new surgeon has recently started performing gender reassignment surgery in the hospital, and his patients have an overnight stay in the PCU following surgery. The nurses on the unit feel unprepared to care for these patients. What is the best initial strategy?

    A. Nursing research council performs a literature review

    B. Nursing education council provides an in-service

    C. Ask the hospital nursing practice council for assistance

    D. Invite the surgeon to provide education to the group

71. A patient has been in the PCU for 5 days being treated for sepsis secondary to a urinary tract infection. The patient presents with an acute change in attention, perception, and memory impairment. This would be most accurately diagnosed as:

    A. Dementia

    B. Delirium

    C. Delirium tremors

    D. Attention-deficit-hyperactivity disorder (ADHD)

72. You administer 30 ml/kg of normal saline & broad spectrum antibiotics to a patient with severe sepsis. The repeat lactate is 3.8 mmol/L. VS: HR 102, RR 24, BP 102/50 (59), T 38.4 C. What should you anticipate next?

    A. Administration of additional IV fluids followed by a repeat lactate

    B. Administration of Norepinephrine infusion and transfer to the ICU

    C. Administration of colloids

    D. Additional broad spectrum antibiotic coverage

73. A 62-year-old female was being treated for pneumonia for 5 days and has now developed dyspnea and tachypnea requiring emergent intubation and mechanical ventilation on your unit. Her chest x-ray reveals bilateral patchy infiltrates with multiple areas of consolidation. Crackles are auscultated throughout her lung fields and she is now requiring 100% FiO_2. A recent ABG reveals a PaO_2 of 48 mm Hg. Which of the following conditions do you suspect the patient has developed?

    A. Status Asthmaticus

    B. Acute Respiratory Distress Syndrome (ARDS)

    C. Acute pulmonary embolism (PE)

    D. Chronic Obstruction Pulmonary Disease (COPD)

74. The Rapid Response Team is activated for a patient decompensating on the PCU with severe shortness of breath. The patient is 2 days status-post myocardial infarction (MI) with PCI. She is diaphoretic with coarse crackles auscultated in bilateral lower lobes.

Patient data is as follows:

BP 90/60 (70)

HR 134

RR 40

T 99.3°F (37.4°C)

O_2 Sat 88% on 10 L simple face mask

pH 7.28

$PaCO_2$ 66

PaO_2 58

HCO_3 22

Based on assessment findings and the ABG results, which of the following treatments do you anticipate?

A. Endotracheal intubation & Lasix 20 mg IV

B. Lasix 20 mg IV & CPAP

C. Stat 12 Lead ECG & metoprolol 5 mg x 1

D. 500 ml (0.9%) normal saline bolus IV & digoxin 0.125 mg IV

75. A patient admitted in hypertensive crisis is assessed for sudden onset right upper extremity weakness, left facial droop, and compliant of 10/10 headache pain. The nurse anticipates which of the following orders?

 A. Administer rtPA and 50 mg IV x 1

 B. Obtain ECG and administer metoprolol 5 mg IV x 1

 C. STAT CT scan head and neck without IV contrast

 D. Administer Morphine 2 mg IV x 1 and reassess pain level in 15 minutes

76. A patient has a long history of unstable angina and complains of chest pain. What is the most concerning finding?

 A. Diaphoresis

 B. Elevated cardiac markers

 C. Shortness of breath

 D. ST elevation

77. The first intervention in a patient with symptoms consistent with hypoglycemia would be:

 A. Administer 1 amp of D_{50}

 B. Administer glucagon IM

 C. Assess the blood glucose level

 D. Administer an IV with D_5W

78. You find your patient lethargic and pale with cool extremities. His HR is 105, BP 100/55, MAP 65 mm Hg, temperature 104° F (40° C) and RR 22. You notice he has blood oozing from old puncture sites, blood tinged urine in the drainage bag, and is coughing up blood tinged sputum. You suspect sepsis induced DIC. What intervention will have the greatest impact on the patient's mortality?

A. Antibiotics

B. Packed red blood cells

C. Low dose heparin

D. Vasoactive agents

79. A 42-year-old male with acute coronary syndrome underwent percutaneous coronary intervention and is being discharged from your unit. You want to educate him on modifiable risk factors. Which of the following topics will you emphasize?

A. Age and exercise

B. Diabetes management and age

C. Hypertension and gender

D. Smoking cessation and hypertension management

80. Which of the following diagnoses describes pulmonary hypertension that results from vasoconstriction of blood vessels leading to and within the pulmonary circulation?

A. Hypoxic pulmonary hypertension

B. Venous pulmonary hypertension

C. Pulmonary arterial hypertension

D. Thromboembolic pulmonary hypertension

81. The family of a comatose man does not want to let the patient's friends and significant other visit. The nurse's best response is to:

    A. Allow the friends and partner to visit when the family is not present

    B. Inform the friends that they will not be able to visit

    C. Initiate a family conference with social work to discuss the issues

    D. Inform the family that they cannot block others from visiting

82. A 68-year-old female is admitted with a diagnosis of acute ischemic stroke. While performing a dysphagia screen, the nurse notices that the patient clears her throat immediately afterward. There is no hacking cough or hoarseness to her voice. The nurse has oral medications to administer. What is the next appropriate action?

    A. Administer the medications and tell the patient to place them on her unaffected side to facilitate swallowing

    B. Insert a nasogastric tube for medication administration

    C. Notify the physician to change the medication administration route to IV instead of by mouth

    D. Request a swallow evaluation and do not administer anything by mouth

83. A 58-year-old admitted with septic shock. The shock has resolved and he is now off vasopressors and inotropic support and has transferred to the PCU. He becomes confused and tries to get out of bed. What type of screening should you assess?

A. CIWA scale for alcohol withdrawal

B. Sepsis screening for severe sepsis

C. CAM assessment for delirium

D. Lactate level for perfusion

84. When monitoring a patient who has been receiving an intravenous heparin infusion for 14 days, the RN notes a sudden decrease in platelets and suspects Type 2 Heparin Induced Thrombocytopenia (HIT). The RN should carefully assess for which of the following?

A. Symptoms of venous thrombosis

B. Pulsus paradoxus

C. Ecchymosis and petechiae

D. Symptoms of internal bleeding

85. The nurse is caring for a patient admitted with severe, stabbing mid-epigastric pain, nausea, vomiting, and rebound tenderness. Patient laboratory data are as follows:

Na^+ 130 mEq/L

K^+ 3.2 mEq/L

Creatinine 1.5 mg/dl

Mg^{++} 1.2 mg/dl

Amylase 130 IU/L

Lipase 55 IU/dl

What order should be anticipated based on the presumed diagnosis?

    A. 1 L normal saline IV bolus and normal saline at 250 ml/hour

    B. D₅W at 100 ml/hour

    C. Regular insulin sliding scale SubQ every six hours

    D. Transfuse 2 units PRBCs

86. You are the leader of a code team resuscitating a 40-year-old female patient who experienced cardiac arrest associated with an acute MI. After 2 minutes of chest compressions & the administration of 1 mg of Epinephrine, the rhythm is reassessed and you see the following on the monitor:

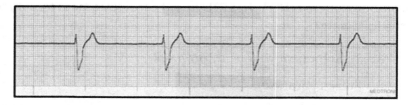

What is your next action?

    A. Administer epinephrine 1 mg IVP

    B. Administer atropine 1 mg IVP

    C. Quickly assess for a pulse

    D. Synchronized cardioversion

87. A focal or diffuse inflammation of the cardiac muscle is known as:

    A. Endocarditis

    B. Pericarditis

    C. Myocarditis

    D. Myocardial infarction

88. Which of the following complications would the nurse assess for after an arteriogram?

    A. Impaired renal function

    B. Acid-base imbalance

    C. Elevated liver enzymes

    D. Increased mean arterial pressure

89. A patient is admitted with a large frontal subdural hematoma. Frontal head injury behaviors include which of the following?

    A. Impulsivity

    B. Language deficits

    C. Visual changes

    D. Unilateral motor deficits

90. Interpret the following arterial blood gas:

    pH 7.50 / $PaCO_2$ 28 / PaO_2 83 / HCO_3 24

    A. Uncompensated metabolic alkalosis with mild hypoxia

    B. Uncompensated respiratory alkalosis with normal oxygenation

    C. Partially compensated metabolic alkalosis with normal oxygenation

    D. Partially compensated respiratory alkalosis with mild hypoxia

91. A nurse working in a high intensity unit has noticed a high stress level in staff impacting relationship establishment with patients and families. What is the appropriate next step for the nurse?

A. Tell the manager the concerns and ask how they will fix it

B. Contact the chair of the practice council & request to add this topic to the agenda.

C. Tell staff about counseling services available through employee assistance

D. Report it the organization compliance department

92. The nurse is caring for patient who is two weeks status post liver transplant. The hospital course has been complicated by acute kidney injury and blood stream infection. The patient has been receiving standard medication therapy for the last five days. On assessment the nurse notices tremors with the extremities at rest and a new petechial rash over the anterior chest and upper extremities. The nurse suspects which complication?

A. Tacrolimus toxicity

B. Thrombocytopenia

C. Acute rejection

D. Liver failure

93. A 73-year-old female is on warfarin therapy for chronic atrial fibrillation. She is scheduled to have a mitral valve replacement for mitral stenosis next week. What advice should the nurse give in regards to her warfarin dosing prior to surgery?

    A. Stop warfarin 4–5 days before surgery

    B. Stop warfarin on the day of surgery

    C. Continue warfarin therapy without interruption

    D. Discontinue warfarin 4–5 days prior to surgery, admission into hospital to place on IV heparin, then stop heparin 4–6 hours prior to surgery

94. A patient has been in the progressive care unit for 2 days s/p thoracotomy for lung cancer. He becomes upset, irritated & restless, kicking and attempting to get out of bed. The Confusion Assessment Method (CAM) is performed and the patient tests positive. Nursing interventions to consider include:

    A. Using a non-opioid scheduled pain protocol

    B. Administering zolpidem (Ambien) 5 mg for sleep

    C. Initiating a waist restraint for safety

    D. Waiting until the patient is calm to reorient him

95. A 58-year-old female experienced an anterior wall MI 2 days ago. She is now c/o chest pain and dizziness. Upon auscultation you note a new, loud systolic murmur. What do you suspect may be the issue?

    A. Acute mitral stenosis

    B. Acute aortic stenosis

    C. Left ventricular outflow obstruction

    D. Acute papillary muscle dysfunction

96. The nurse is precepting a new graduate nurse in the care of a patient immediately status post small bowel resection. The nurse states that if tachycardia, tachypnea, or left shoulder pain is assessed, the provider needs to be called immediately. The new graduate nurse understands these symptoms could demonstrate which complication?

    A. Pulmonary Embolism

    B. Anastomotic leak

    C. Myocardial infarction

    D. Atelectasis

97. A patient is admitted for airway monitoring following a self-inflicted stab wound to the neck. The patient arrives in four-point locked restraints from the ED. What is the appropriate priority for the nurse?

    A. Verify placement of IV sites

    B. Palpate distal pulses in all extremities

    C. Perform a nurse bedside swallow screen

    D. Assess & documentation a suicide risk screen

98. Which set of lab values is commonly seen in acute pancreatitis?

    A. Hyperglycemia, hypercalcemia, hyperkalemia

    B. Hyperglycemia, hypocalcemia, hypokalemia

    C. Hypoglycemia, hypocalcemia, hypokalemia

    D. Hypoglycemia, hypercalcemia, hyperkalemia

99. A patient admitted to the PCU with seizures refractory to his current home medications. He is started on Depakote (Valproic acid). The patient has a central line and urinary catheter in place. Which action by the nurse demonstrates an understanding of medication side effects?

A. Collaborate daily with the medical team to evaluate the need of the central line and urinary catheter

B. Order seizure pads from central supply

C. Apply sequential compression devices upon arrival to the unit

D. Advocate for daily bowel care protocol

100. You are caring for a patient in Diabetic Ketoacidosis (DKA). The resident requests to be notified once the anion gap closes. Which components from serum lab values are used to determine the anion gap?

A. BUN, sodium, potassium, magnesium

B. Sodium, glucose, BUN, potassium

C. Creatinine, sodium, chloride, magnesium

D. Sodium, potassium, chloride, bicarbonate

101. A common laboratory finding in a patient with diabetes insipidus is:

A. Decreased serum osmolality

B. Decreased urine output

C. Elevated urine specific gravity

D. Elevated serum osmolality

102. Long term medical management of heart failure includes which of the following?

   A. Beta blockers, ACE inhibitors & aldosterone antagonists

   B. ACE inhibitors, ARBs and vasopressors

   C. ARBs, beta blockers & calcium channel blockers

   D. Vasopressors, ACE inhibitors & calcium channel blockers

103. The nurse is monitoring a patient status post epicardial pacing wire removal. The hospital protocol requires assessment for signs and symptoms of Beck's Triad with each vital sign evaluation. The nurse understands the risk to the patient is:

   A. Pleural effusion

   B. Cerebral swelling

   C. Pulmonary embolism

   D. Cardiac tamponade

104. The nurse is caring for a patient status post aortic valve replacement (AVR) and epicardial pacing wire removal. Six hours after the epicardial wires are removed patient data is as follows:

   HR 150

   BP 88/78 (81)

   Jugular venous distention (+ JVD)

   Mottled knees

The patient is clinically assessed and is diaphoretic, difficult to arouse with thready and weak peripheral pulses and distant heart tones. These findings are most indicative of:

A. Pulmonary embolism

B. Acute papillary muscle rupture

C. Cardiac tamponade

D. Septic shock

105. An elderly patient with dementia has a new diagnosis of carotid artery stenosis following transient ischemic attack. Which statement by the family demonstrates good understanding of teaching?

A. "We will plan for a low sodium diet"

B. "We will call 911 for any signs of stroke"

C. "We will help avoid any strenuous exercise"

D. "We will stop giving blood pressure medication"

106. A 45-year-old patient returned to the PCU following a right pneumonectomy 8 hours ago. Her oxygen saturation has been steady at 95% on 40% FiO_2, but has begun slowly dropping in the last 10 minutes and is now 90%. The nurse's initial response is to:

A. Position the patient with the right side down

B. Increase the FiO_2 to 60%

C. Position the patient with the left side down

D. Draw an arterial blood gas to assess ventilation

107. The presence of a U wave on the electrocardiogram is associated with which electrolyte disturbance?

  A. Hyperkalemia

  B. Hypokalemia

  C. Hypercalcemia

  D. Hypocalcemia

108. You are caring for a Native American patient with end stage heart failure who is not expected to survive this hospitalization. His tribal leaders would like to be present during his passing and would like to conduct tribal songs and customs prior to his death. They expect about 30 people to be present for the ceremony. What would be your best action for this request?

  A. Tell them 30 people is unreasonable and to prioritize the list

  B. Move the patient to a bigger room and allow the ceremony to proceed as long as the environment is safe

  C. Tell the group this is an unreasonable request

  D. Suggest they reconsider and alter the ceremony to keep the room quiet

109. The nurse is caring for a patient with resolving cerebral artery vasospasm after a ruptured aneurysm. Nimodipine 60 mg PO is due to be administered. Patient data is as follows:

BP 92/68 (76)

HR 98

RR 16

Which is the appropriate next step for the nurse?

A. Hold the Nimodipine, document SBP

B. Contact the provider for additional orders

C. Administer Nimodipine 30 mg PO and reevaluate the SBP in 30 minutes

D. Hold Nimodipine and reevaluate SBP in 30 minutes

110. **The nurse is caring for a patient 3 days post liver transplant. Initially, the post-operative blood glucose was 221 mg/dL, requiring a continuous insulin infusion. The nurse understands monitoring the blood glucose frequently is indicated for assessment of:**

A. Surgical site infection

B. Urinary tract infection

C. Hepatorenal syndrome

D. Acute liver failure

111. **The most common cause of death after a myocardial infarction is:**

A. Ventricular septal defect

B. Cardiogenic shock

C. Dysrhythmias

D. Heart failure

112. A patient with an anterior wall MI should be monitored for which of the following complications?

A. Right BBB & 2nd degree Type 2 heart block

B. 1st degree heart block

C. Aberrantly conducted rhythms

D. Supraventricular tachycardia

113. Which nursing diagnosis is of priority in a patient with acute pancreatitis?

A. Fluid volume deficit

B. Ineffective airway clearance

C. Knowledge deficit

D. Potential for infection

114. The rationale for using Dobutamine in decompensated heart failure is to:

A. Decrease myocardial ischemia

B. Improve urine output

C. Improve myocardial contraction

D. Decrease oxygen consumption

115. A patient with newly diagnosed dementia was admitted to the PCU after an accidental metoprolol overdose. The patient has a HR of 42. What medication would you expect the provider to order as an antidote?

A. Flumazenil

B. Glucagon hydrochloride

C. Naltrexone hydrochloride

D. Deferoxamine mesylate

116. Your patient shares with you that they are not comfortable going to the general floor after you informed them that they are transferring to the general medical unit. What is the most holistic response?

A. "Don't worry, I know that they will take great care of you on the unit."

B. "Do you recognize this means you are doing much better and are able to go home soon?"

C. "Tell me more about concerns you have regarding the transfer."

D. "Sorry, but it's the doctor's orders."

117. Your patient is receiving a RBC transfusion secondary to bleeding with a hematocrit of 20. Ten minutes into the transfusion the patient complaining of shortness of breath and chest pain. Which of the following actions should you take?

A. Apply oxygen and call for a 12-lead ECG

B. Call for a stat chest x-ray as she may have a pulmonary embolus

C. Elevate the head of the bed and give a saline bolus

D. Immediately stop the transfusion and recheck vital signs

118. The nurse has expressed concern to the advanced practice provider that a patient on hospital day two admitted for a left-sided intra-ventricular hemorrhage is experiencing an extension of the initial hemorrhage. Which of the following assessment findings would confirm this suspicion?

A. Left pupil greater than right and non-reactive with noted right upper extremity extensor posturing

B. Left Hand grasp weakness with numbness and tingling

C. Right pupil greater than left and non-reactive with noted left upper extremity extensor posturing

D. 8/10 headache pain unrelieved by Tylenol

119. A patient with pulmonary arterial hypertension is on an intravenous Epoprostenol (Flolan) infusion and experiences a sudden onset of cough and hemoptysis. The nurse notes increased work of breathing and the following vital signs: HR 130, BP 95/60 (72), O_2 sat 85% on 2 L O_2 and pain 6/10 in the center of the chest. Which diagnostic test should be anticipated at this point?

A. Chest radiography to rule out pneumonia

B. Computed tomography with contrast to rule out pulmonary embolism

C. Echocardiogram to assess the patient's ejection fraction

D. Cardiac biomarkers to rule out myocardial infarction

120. A patient is admitted with adrenal insufficiency. The provider orders Dexamethasone (Decadron). Which side effect should you anticipate?

    A. Increased potassium level

    B. Increased calcium level

    C. Hypoglycemia

    D. Proximal muscle weakness

121. Which of the following is most likely the cause of a systolic murmur auscultated at the right sternal border, 2nd ICS?

    A. Mitral stenosis

    B. Aortic stenosis

    C. Mitral insufficiency

    D. Aortic insufficiency

122. Clinical signs of cardiogenic shock secondary to acute left ventricular failure include:

    A. Hypotension, S_4 heart sound, pericardial friction rub

    B. S_3 heart sound, Hypotension, systolic murmur

    C. Diastolic murmur, S_4 heart sound, Hypertension

    D. Crackles, S_3 heart sound, hypotension

123. Which of the following antipsychotic medications has the least effect on the QT interval?

    A. Seroquel (quetiapine)

    B. Haldol (haloperidol)

    C. Droperidol (inapsine)

    D. Abilify (aripiprazole)

124. A 72-year-old male is recovering in the PCU after a myocardial infarction. According to Erickson, which task is appropriate to maintain for an older adult?

    A. Maintaining unity with spouse/partner

    B. Examining personal assets

    C. Maintaining a sense of self-worth

    D. Participating in organizations

125. The nurse is caring for a patient with a history of chronic kidney disease who was admitted to the hospital for inpatient dialysis prior to placement of an arteriovenous fistula. Which of the following ECG changes would be most alarming?

    A. Tall, peaked T waves

    B. Shortened QT segment

    C. Inverted T waves

    D. Elevated ST segment

You can do it!

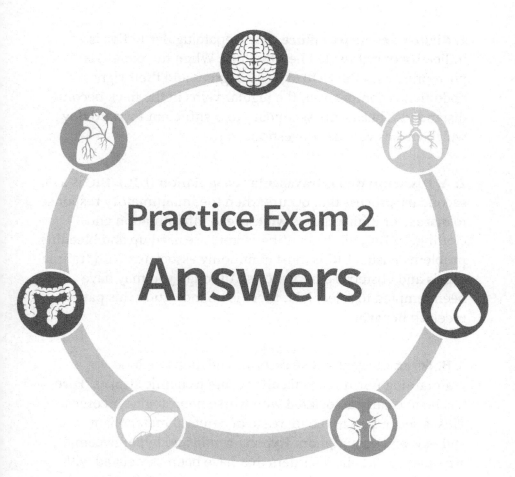

Practice Exam 2
Answers

Practice Exam #2 Answers with rationales

1. **Right-sided heart failure.** The Hepatojugular Reflex is indicative of right-sided heart failure. When the patient is positioned with the HOB at 30-45 degrees and their right abdomen is compressed, the jugular veins in the neck become distended. This occurs secondary to insufficient forward flow, which causes venous congestion.

2. **A. Disseminated intravascular coagulation (DIC).** DIC is a secondary process that occurs when the inflammatory response to disease or injury causes widespread inflammation and clotting. In DIC, all the clotting factors are used up and bleeding problems ensue. DIC is most commonly associated with trauma, sepsis and obstetric emergencies. Although you may have been tempted to select HIT, there is no indication this patient received heparin.

3. **B. Fever.** Current stroke recommendations include maintaining normothermia after acute ischemic strokes. Fever has been clearly associated with worse neurologic outcomes. This is secondary to the increase in cerebral metabolism rate and oxygen consumption. Hyponatremia and hyperglycemia are other metabolic disorders that have been associated with worsening infarcts and neurological outcomes following ischemic strokes.

4. **B. Teach incentive spirometer use.** The patient's vitals are stable; blood pressure is a bit low but the mean arterial pressure is adequate and a permissive hypotension strategy is often used in the presence of solid organ injury. Incentive spirometer use is essential in avoiding further pulmonary complications

such as atelectasis and pneumonia. Pain medication should be considered, but may have slightly sedating effects and should be administered after spirometry if possible.

5. **B. Hypomagnesemia.** It is important to measure QT intervals because of its association with severe ventricular arrhythmias, specifically Torsades de pointes. QT prolongation can be secondary to congenital long QT syndrome, rare genetic disorders, medications such as Quinidine, Sotalol, Amiodarone, Haldol, Seroquel, or electrolyte imbalances such hypomagnesemia, hypokalemia, or hypocalcemia.

6. **A. Discontinue captopril, add losartan (Cozaar) 50 mg daily.** A dry, hacking cough is a common adverse effect of ACE inhibitors such as captopril. When present, the ACE-I can be replaced with an angiotensin II receptor blocker (ARB) such as losartan. This should be the initial medication change, and since there are no other indications of adverse or inadequate effects, the rest of the medications should not be adjusted at this time.

7. **B. Sodium, potassium, chloride, bicarbonate.** The anion gap is the calculated difference between the positively charged ions (sodium and potassium) and the negatively charged ions (chloride and bicarbonate) in the serum. A decreasing anion gap is suggestive of progress of resolution of DKA. You may hear this referred to as "closing the gap". Sodium, glucose, and BUN would be used to assess osmolality. Urine and serum creatinine levels are used to assess renal function, usually as part of a 24-hour creatinine clearance test.

8. **D. Decreased right atrial preload.** In the setting of sepsis, there is a significant inflammatory response. Blood vessels vasodilate and there is significant capillary leak. The combination of these physiologic changes leads to intravascular

volume depletion and decreased preload. Volume resuscitation is a priority when managing patient with severe sepsis and septic shock.

9. **A. Nausea, diarrhea, and shortness of breath**. These signs are commonly seen in an individual with anxiety. Dilated pupils are not correlated with anxiety disorders; however, it may be caused by an overdose of benzodiazepines.

10. **D. Hypertension, peripheral artery disease, diabetes.** A history of high blood pressure, liver or kidney disease, cardiac or abdominal surgery, peripheral arterial disease, and diabetes are risk factors for acute kidney injury.

11. **D. Defibrillation, chest compressions & airway management.** Compressions, defibrillation, airway and breathing (CDAB) is the treatment priority in the case of pulseless ventricular tachycardia or ventricular fibrillation. Beginning chest compressions immediately and defibrillating as soon as possible takes precedence over any medications.

12. **B. Chest x-ray & pulmonary hygiene.** Atelectasis is a risk following major abdominal surgery. The patient has low oxygen saturations on room air is in danger of changes in stability. Starting with a chest x-ray and pulmonary hygiene to open airways and mobilize secretions is the initial place for the nurse to start in the management of this complication.

13. **B. Begin feedings via jejunal route to minimize pancreatic stimulation.** Enteral feedings are preferred. Clinical management has changed from maintaining NPO status and waiting for lab values to return to normal and pain to dissipate. Utilization of jejunal feedings maintain gut integrity and minimize pancreatic stimulation.

14. **C. Perform a focused neurologic exam.** The change in level of consciousness may be indicative of increased intracranial pressure. A focused neurological exam should be performed and compared to baseline data while notifying the provider.

15. **C. Antibiotics.** The major goal of treating metabolic syndrome is to reduce the risk of coronary artery disease and the secondary goal is to treat or prevent the onset of Type II diabetes. Risk factors for metabolic syndrome include hypertension, obesity, elevated fasting glucose or diagnosed Type II diabetes, hyperlipidemia and hypercholesterolemia.

16. **B. Left axis deviation.** Leads I and aVF form the perfect x and y axis to determine direction of electrical axis. If the QRS complex is upright in both leads, axis is normal. Negative deflection in both leads depicts an extreme right axis deviation. Negative QRS deflection in Lead I and positive deflection in Lead aVF are associated with right axis deviation.

17. **B. Diabetic ketoacidosis (DKA).** The key information in this question is the development of ketones which is seen in DKA. This patient has all the symptoms associated with DKA; decreased LOC, tachypnea, likely Kussmaul's breathing, presence of ketones, elevated serum osmolality, acidosis & anion gap. In HHS, ketone production is not seen because Type II diabetes patients have some endogenous insulin.

18. **D. Hyperkalemia.** ACE-inhibitors, angiotensin receptor blockers and aldosterone receptor blockers can potentially impair renal function and their ability to excrete potassium. As a result, serum potassium levels may rise.

19. **D. Partially compensated metabolic acidosis.** The low pH indicates acidosis, and the low bicarb rather than elevated CO_2 indicate a metabolic process. The low CO_2 shows that compensation has begun, so this ABG is a partially compensated (but still alarming) metabolic acidosis.

20. **A. Chvostek sign.** Chvostek sign is a facial twitch elicited by tapping over the facial nerve. A twitch, or positive test, indicates hypocalcemia and should prompt lab work and/or treatment. Kehr's sign is often observed in patients with splenic injury. It is a referred pain to the left shoulder. Kernig's sign is seen in subarachnoid hemorrhage, meningitis and conditions of meningeal irritation. It is considered positive when the thigh is flexed at the hip with the knee at a 90 degree angle; extension in the knee is painful leading to resistance. With Cullen's sign you will see periumbilical ecchymosis. This is often found in the setting of necrotizing pancreatitis, abdominal trauma and aortic rupture.

21. **A. Completion of the Confusion Assessment Method (CAM) and 12 Lead ECG.** The risk of QTc prolongation can contribute to dysrhythmias for a patient already at risk for dysrhythmias after surgery. The priority data to collect is the CAM-ICU (Confusion Assessment Method) assessment to assess for a possible delirium and a 12 Lead ECG to track changes in QTc.

22. **B. Call the OR to get a status report and notify him of the reason for the delay.** Family members need accurate and timely information, particularly during stressful procedures. Ascertaining the cause of delay will help the family member understand the reasons and hopefully help him remain calm.

23. **B. VVI.** Since the patient is generating irregular electrical activity from the atria, the pacer should be set to ignore the

'noise' and instead monitor and pace ventricular activity to sustain the set heart rate. The atria cannot be paced when in atrial fibrillation.

24. **A. Alpha cells.** Beta cells produce insulin. Delta cells produce somatostatin. Kappa cells are not part of the anatomy of the pancreas.

25. **C. Ventricular hypertrophy**. When the ventricles are thickened, as in hypertrophy, it is more difficult to fill them adequately. The atria eject more forcefully, and the vibration of this ejection causes the S_4 heart sound. In the setting of pericarditis, a pericardial friction rub may be auscultated. A S3 heart sound (ventricular gallop) is auscultated in heart failure with fluid overload. A split S1 may be auscultated with a bundle branch block or frequent PVCs.

26. **B. Serum osmolality of 320.** The profound dehydration will lead to an elevated serum osmolality in Diabetes Insipidus because of the water loss. In diabetes insipidus there is a lack of ADH. The sodium level may elevate while the urine specific gravity will drop due to dilutional effects.

27. **D. Gastrointestinal bleeding 2 months ago.** The patient is exhibiting signs of stroke, which is likely to be ischemic. Optimal treatment is administration of recombinant tissue plasminogen activator (rtPA). Contraindications to rtPA include recent history of bleeding (within 3 months), so a patient who experienced recent GI bleeding may not be eligible until the history is clarified. Other bleeding complications or surgeries within the past 3 months (varying by condition) are also contraindications. Since the patient takes a daily aspirin, lab values should be reviewed, but anticoagulant administration is not of itself a contraindication.

28. **B. Decreased level of consciousness.** A change in LOC or mental status is the first sign of problems with a shunt as well as other problems that cause increased ICP. Nystagmus and slurred speech would likely come later, depending on the location of the shunt. Pupil inequality is a late sign of increased ICP and may indicate impending herniation.

29. **B. Hypercapnia.** In acute asthma exacerbation, hypercapnia or elevated $PaCO_2$ is an ominous sign and indicates the patient is becoming fatigued and going into acute respiratory failure.

30. **C. The kidneys are not responding appropriately to vasopressin (ADH).** Diabetes Insipidus (DI) occurs when an individual has a deficiency or insensitivity to vasopressin (ADH). There are three types of DI: neurogenic DI, nephrogenic DI, and Dipsogenic DI. Neurogenic DI occurs when there has been damage to the posterior pituitary resulting in a deficiency of vasopressin. Nephrogenic DI occurs when the kidneys are not adequately responding to vasopressin. Dipsogenic DI occurs when there is excessive ingestion of water, which suppresses vasopressin release, which leads to polyuria. Diabetes Mellitus type 1 occurs from insufficient insulin production by pancreatic beta cells.

31. **D. Cool, pale, moist skin.** Cardiogenic shock results from the impaired ability of the ventricle to pump blood forward, which leads to a decrease in stroke volume (SV) and an increase in left end diastolic volume (LEDV). The decrease in SV activates the RASS system resulting in vasoconstriction, which causes an increase in systemic vasculature resistance. The increase in LEDV results in increased left atrial preload, which manifests as pulmonary congestion and crackles. This pulmonary edema causes impaired gas exchange and impaired tissue perfusion resulting in cool, pale, moist skin. You would not expect to hear wheezes with pulmonary edema. This would be more common in a restrictive airway disease.

32. **C. Norepinephrine.** The Surviving Sepsis Guidelines recommend Norepinephrine (Levophed) as the first line vasopressor for hypotension that is no longer responsive to fluids. Norepinephrine has mostly alpha receptor innervation and increases the blood pressure & MAP through vasoconstriction without affecting HR or stroke volume. Dobutamine is a positive inotrope that will increase CO and decrease afterload, which can worsen hypotension, therefore it is not recommended as the first line therapy for hypotension. Dopamine increases CO and MAP, but it has significant tachyarrhythmia effects on the heart and increases myocardial oxygen demands. Vasopressin is a potent vasoconstrictor that has been found effective in refractory hypotension, but is not the first line drug therapy for hypotension in septic shock.

33. **C. Email the unit practice council chair and ask to have this added to the next meeting agenda.** Bringing this concern to the unit practice council is appropriate. Through the determination of the practice council it would be found as a resource for dissemination of possible new practices. The practice council would be an opportunity to review best practices, standards of practice, and get buy in from other staff members to lead the change.

34. **B. Lactated ringers at 100 ml/hour 12 hours before and after the procedure.** Mucomyst is often prescribed to prevent contrast induced nephropathy. The dose is usually 600 mg PO every 12 hours x 4 doses. However, the evidence doesn't fully support Mucomyst. Furosemide and Mannitol will not protect the kidneys from the effects of the contrast material. Intravenous fluids keep the kidneys flushed to prevent renal tubule damage from contrast material.

35. **A. "Percutaneous coronary intervention is the best therapy for MI."** PCI is the evidence-based gold standard of care for

acute coronary syndrome. Once the infarct is determined to involve ST elevation (STEMI or STE-ACS) or no ST elevation (NSTEMI or NSTE-ACS), duration of symptoms and history of bleeding will help determine the optimal treatment for that patient. If required, PCI should ideally be completed within 90 minutes for STEMI and 24 hours for NSTE-ACS. If it is not possible to get the patient to the Cath lab within 90–120 min for STEMI, fibrinolytics should be considered. Lab work provides important evidence, but the 12 Lead ECG is essential for determining treatment.

36. **A. Nasogastric tubes.** With a basilar skull fracture, improper insertion of an NG tube can result in cannulation of the brain. Insertion of any type of tube (NG, feeding, suction) should be avoided or performed by a provider using fluoroscopy.

37. **A. Metoprolol.** Beta-blockers help by slowing the heart rate to maximize diastolic filling time. In addition, beta blockers decrease myocardial oxygen consumption by decreasing contractility. Diuretics decrease cardiac output by decreasing filling pressures in the hypertrophic ventricles. Inotropes, and vasodilators are typically used in dilated cardiomyopathy to strengthen contractions and control fluid volumes; in hypertrophic cardiomyopathy they may contribute to left ventricular outflow obstruction.

38. **B. Dilutional hyponatremia.** This is a classic case of dilutional hyponatremia often caused by SIADH or Syndrome of inappropriate anti-diuretic hormone. There is an excess of ADH causing the kidneys to hold on to water thereby diluting the serum sodium levels. Diabetes insipidus has the opposite symptoms due to a lack of ADH. Patients develop profound urine (water) loss causing increased sodium levels and serum osmolality.

39. **A. Urinary output, lactate, ScvO$_2$.** Urinary output, lactate & ScvO$_2$ are parameters to assess end organ perfusion. In the setting of poor perfusion, the urine output will be low, venous or arterial lactate will be elevated and the ScvO$_2$ will be low. A common target ScvO$_2$ in the setting of shock is > 70%. A 12 Lead ECG gives a picture of the electrical conduction of the heart and will identify ischemia, which can result in poor end organ perfusion, but is not valuable as an estimate of perfusion.

40. **B. Cultural norms for pain expression.** It is important to continuality learn about cultures of the patients you care for without assuming the patient adheres to these beliefs or follows the behavior most common to that culture. It is important to ask the patient how they feel about expressing pain and what their pain level expectations are. Take time to develop a plan for managing their pain. Some cultures may find using the faces on the pain scale demeaning. Disregarding the patient's culture, ethnicity, religion, and beliefs is not appropriate as the nurse must care for not only the physical, but also psychosocial health and well-being of the patient.

41. **C. Aortic stenosis.** The stiff aorta causes increased noise during systole and impairs outflow, leading to pulmonary edema and rales. Mitral stenosis causes an apical diastolic murmur; mitral regurgitation causes a holosystolic murmur with split S2, and aortic regurgitation leads to a high pitched decrescendo diastolic murmur.

42. **A. Petechiae.** Thrombocytopenia is a condition in which the number of platelets available to assist with coagulation is inadequate, which increases the patient's risk of hemorrhage. Superficial bleeding occurs under the skin and appears as a reddish-purple pinpoint sized rash or spots. Other signs of thrombocytopenia include unexplained bleeding from gums or

nose, easy or excessive bruising (purpura), prolonged bleeding times, blood in urine or stool, fatigue, enlarged spleen, or jaundice.

43. **A. Dumping syndrome.** 10–50% of gastrointestinal surgeries result in some form of dumping syndrome. This condition is also known as rapid gastric emptying, as it is characterized by rapid emptying of the stomach contents into the small intestine. This occurs when food, especially sugar, moves from the stomach to the small bowel too quickly. This leads to large amounts of undigested food entering the small intestine and increased propulsive motility, which results in loss of nutrients and impaired bowel function. Acute renal failure, diabetes mellitus, and pancreatitis are not common complications from gastrointestinal surgery.

44. **C. Unfractionated heparin with daily PTT, adding Coumadin after 1–2 days.** In a stable patient with a PE, heparin is used to prevent the clot from further growth, allowing the body to break it down normally. Coumadin (warfarin) therapy is used long term for anticoagulation.

45. **B. Preform a literature review to determine best practice.** Professionalism involves mentoring others. The preceptor is mentoring and teaching the orientee, but the preceptor must also be open to learn from the orientee. If there is a difference in methods for performing a specific task, the best approach is to perform a literature review to determine best practice. Stating that the orientee is wrong, without rationale or evidence-based research, does not acknowledge the skills and knowledge the orientee is bringing to the team. Surveying other nurses can be done, but may not result in the latest evidence-based approach. Ignoring the difference and assuming that the orientee knows does not promote growth or best practice in either the preceptor or orientee.

46. A. Call for help and safely guide the patient to the floor. Patient safety is the first priority. Once the patient is safe from immediate harm or injury, the seizure activity must be terminated. Seizure abatement is accomplished by the administration of a benzodiazepine. Anti-epileptics are useful in the prevention of seizure of activity.

47. C. Notify the provider of a potential anastomotic leak. Potential complications of bariatric surgery include infection and bleeding, and gastric bypass also carries the risk of anastomotic leak. Signs may be insidious such that elevated heart rate is the only indicator before sepsis begins. CT scan can confirm the leak, but early recognition and treatment is crucial in achieving a good outcome. The patient may need a sepsis protocol and fluid administration, but the provider needs to be aware of the symptoms right away.

48. D. Reduced renal perfusion pressure. The release of renin from the juxtaglomerular cells is stimulated by reduced glomerular pressure at the afferent arteriole. Hyponatremia and reduced left ventricular end diastolic pressure may result in reduced renal perfusion pressure, but these two alone do not cause the release of renin. Reduced cerebral perfusion pressure initiates cerebral vasodilatation.

49. B. Infero-posterior. Leads II, III, and aVF assess the inferior wall of the left ventricle. The right coronary artery (RCA) is of issue. In about 90% of the population, the RCA also supplies blood to the posterior wall. Injury to this area manifests itself with ST-depression in the septal leads with a large R-wave in lead V_2 which is a reciprocal change. In this scenario, visually flipping leads V_1 and V_2 180 degrees on its horizontal axis will reveals ST-elevation with pathologic Q-waves.

50. **D. Mitral stenosis.** The mitral valve is open during diastole on the S_2 sound. Hearing a murmur at the mitral auscultation site during diastole results from a narrow opening in the valve. Aortic murmurs are auscultated loudest at the right sternal border, 2nd intercostal space.

51. **D. Ischemic stroke.** Patients with HIT may develop systemic thrombosis. Patients with HIT need to be routinely evaluated for development of a DVT, pulmonary embolism, stroke, myocardial infarction, or renal impairment.

52. **A. Creatinine 2.8 mg/dL.** Vancomycin has a high risk of nephrotoxicity and an elevated serum creatinine is important to review with the providers to ensure the plan will be to continue to the planned medication treatment.

53. **C. Left pupil greater than right and minimally reactive.** Assessment manifestations for cerebral insults including head bleeds and ischemic events include ipsilateral pupil changes and contralateral motor extremity changes.

54. **C. Chest tube insertion.** When a patient displays hemodynamic instability or becomes unstable secondary to a pneumothorax, the American Association of Chest Physicians recommends emergent treatment with chest tube insertion. Oxygen administration of 3 L/min or higher is also recommended to correct hypoxemia and is associated with an increase in air reabsorption when compared with room air alone.

The goal in treating pneumothorax is to relieve the air that is trapped in the pleural space and causing pressure. Medications may be necessary to treat a pulmonary disorder that causes the pneumothorax, but not one secondary to central line placement. An echocardiogram would be helpful if a tension pneumothorax or tamponade was suspected to be the cause of the hemodynamic instability, but would not take priority over a chest tube insertion.

55. A. Decreased urine osmolality. ATN is a type of intrarenal failure, in which during the diuretic phase the kidneys lose the ability to concentrate urine, which causes a decrease in urine osmolality and specific gravity resulting in dilute urine. The kidneys also lose the ability to reabsorb sodium, resulting in a high urine sodium level. In renal failure hyperphosphatemia is often observed.

56. A. Systolic murmur. The mitral valve is closed during systole so that blood can be ejected from the left ventricle into the body. Failure of the valve to close completely results in blood being pushed from the LV backward into the left atrium, causing a murmur during systole.

57. C. Grey-Turner's sign; retroperitoneal bleed. Bruising in the lower abdomen and flank region is known as Grey-Turner's sign. It is indicative of retroperitoneal bleeding and warrants imaging for further diagnosis. Kernig's sign is observed when the patient cannot fully extend the knee when the hip is flexed and is indicative of meningitis. Cullen's sign is superficial edema and ecchymosis in the subcutaneous fatty tissue around the umbilicus and is indicative of intra-abdominal bleeding. Brudzinski's sign is when the passive flexion of the neck causes flexion of both legs and thighs and is indicative of meningitis.

58. D. Furosemide. Loop diuretics, like furosemide, inhibit the reabsorption of sodium, potassium, calcium, and magnesium in the loop of Henle. Furosemide is used to treat pulmonary edema and has an added benefit of lowering the calcium levels. Spironolactone is a weak diuretic that primarily targets the distal nephron, where only small amounts of sodium is reabsorbed. It is usually combined with other diuretics to increase efficacy. Mannitol is a diuretic usually to remove excess body water in certain kidney conditions, reducing swelling of the brain or reducing intraocular pressure.

59. **B. HR 45 bpm.** Bradycardia is the best indicator that shock is from a neurogenic cause such as spinal shock. A low cardiac output and hypotension are consistent across shock states. Neurogenic and other forms of distributive shock result in decreased afterload rather than elevated afterload.

60. **D. Correcting her fluid deficit.** Patients with DKA have a profound fluid deficit. Correcting the deficit is of high priority as it may lead to hemodynamic compromise. Glucose levels will start to fall as fluids & insulin are administered. Insulin will push potassium into the cell causing a drop in serum potassium levels.

61. **A. ARDS, DIC, and hypovolemic shock.** The sequelae of SIRS produces pulmonary complications due to the proximity of structures. Capillary leakage at the alveolar capillary level predisposes the patient to ARDS. Initiation of the inflammatory response also activates the clotting cascade. If left untreated, all clotting factors are consumed resulting in DIC. Fluid volume deficit from and bleeding associated with DIC results in hypovolemic shock. Thrombotic disorders are possible but not seen as commonly as ARDS, DIC, and hypovolemic shock. Tension pneumothorax and chylothorax have no physiological basis. Liver and renal failure are directly associated with hypoperfusion and shock as opposed to pancreatitis.

62. **A. Voice hoarseness.** In a patient with multiple bee stings, you should be monitoring for signs of anaphylaxis. Voice hoarseness can be a sign of laryngeal edema, a manifestation

of anaphylactic shock. Tachycardia, not bradycardia, is a sign of anaphylaxis. You should be concerned with an elevated WBC and temperature as these could indicate infection, which could lead to sepsis, but they are not indicators of anaphylaxis.

63. **D. Glycopyrrolate (Robinul).** Glycopyrrolate is an anti-adrenergic that decreases secretions and is part of the medical management of respiratory failure in a patient with chronic pulmonary disease. Anxiolytics should be used with caution as they may increase sedation and worsen pulmonary status. Subcutaneous epinephrine is not appropriate for patients with heart conditions and theophylline is also not the preferred management. Other medications will include albuterol (Ventolin), ipratropium bromide (Atrovent) and steroids.

64. **A. Positive inotropic agents, diuretics & vasodilators.** Acute exacerbations of heart failure involve fluid overload of an already taxed heart. Vasodilation helps decrease preload and afterload, and positive inotropes help with contractility, so cardiac output is improved in multiple ways. Beta blockers should be used cautiously or held if the patient is hypotensive because of negative inotropic effects.

65. **D. Pericarditis.** Inflammation of the pericardium is not uncommon following bypass surgery. Chest pain that is relieved with positioning is typically pleuritic pain, and is common in conditions causing cardiac inflammation.

66. **C. Prevent thrombus formation.** Early anticoagulation, sometimes < 1 day postop, is indicated for patients with valve replacement surgery. Prior to the 48 hour mark, a patient should be hemodynamically stable and may or may not be receiving antibiotics. Monitoring for conduction disturbances also remains a priority.

67. B. Decreased platelets, decreased fibrinogen, increased D-dimer. In a bleeding patient, coagulation factors are expected to be lower than normal. D-dimer is produced when plasmin breaks apart clots, and is indicative of a current clotting problem.

68. C. Seizure activity with onset of stroke symptoms. Thrombolytic therapy using rtPA is the most common treatment for ischemic stroke, provided the patient meets the inclusion/exclusion criterion. The inclusion criteria includes: patient is over the age of 18, less than 3 hours since the onset of stroke symptoms, and a clinical diagnosis and CT scan verifying ischemic stroke. Exclusion criteria includes: occurrence of a seizure at onset of the stroke, major surgery or trauma in the past two weeks, or a stroke or traumatic brain injury in the last 3 months.

69. D. Volume resuscitation. The patient is experiencing a major fluid volume deficit from an osmotic diuresis due to hyperglycemia. Initial volume resuscitation with an isotonic fluid is imperative. When the glucose is lowered to about 250, a dextrose source should be added to the IV solution.

70. D. Invite the surgeon to provide education to the group. Inviting the surgeon not only provides information on the physiological and psychosocial needs of transgender patients, but also promotes collaboration, facilitation of learning, and builds relationship between the provider and the unit. Literature review and in-service should also be explored, and the nursing practice council should be involved so that other units who care for these patients can also be educated.

71. B. Delirium. Delirium is an acute disorder characterized by inattention, alterations in perception, disorganized thinking and memory impairment. It is often a symptom of an underlying condition such as acute infection, medication overdose, substance intoxication, electrolyte disorders, or dehydration. Delirium tremors are associated with alcohol withdrawal and are usually accompanied by tremors, diaphoresis, anorexia, nausea and/or vomiting, increased HR and RR, agitation, and visual or auditory hallucinations. ADHD is associated with symptoms of limited attention and hyperactivity. Patients most commonly experience excitability, impulsivity, irritability, difficulty focusing, short attention span, and may display mood swings.

72. **A. Administration of additional IV fluids and insertion of a central line.** An elevated repeat lactate indicates inadequate fluid resuscitation, especially when combined with ongoing tachycardia and hypotension. The lactate level should be repeated after the fluid bolus. Ideally the lactate will decrease or clear. The goal is to normalize the lactate.

73. **B. Acute Respiratory Distress Syndrome (ARDS).** ARDS is an inflammatory syndrome marked by the disruption of the alveolar-capillary membrane resulting in increased capillary membrane permeability, which allows leakage of fluid and protein into the pulmonary interstitium. This results in clinical manifestations of dyspnea and tachypnea.

The 2012 Berlin Criteria defined ARDS as a PaO_2/FiO_2 ratio less than or equal to 300 mm Hg with bilateral infiltrates on chest radiography and refractory hypoxemia. Mild ARDS is defined as a P/F ratio < 300, moderate ARDS P/F ratio < 200, severe ARDS < 100.   In ARDS there is usually an inflammatory process that predisposes a patient. In this case pneumonia was the insult that put the patient at risk of developing ARDS. Status Asthmaticus, acute PE and COPD may present with dyspnea and tachypnea, but not with bilateral infiltrates and crackles.

74. **A. Endotracheal intubation & Lasix 20 mg IV.** While the patient is demonstrating a fluid overload state, the ABG shows acute respiratory failure with respiratory acidosis. The registered nurse should anticipate endotracheal intubation urgently as a priority intervention as well as administration of loop diuretics. If the patient is alert, Bi-Pap may also be considered for ventilatory support to bridge the patient to prevent intubation. CPAP will not likely provide adequate ventilatory support.

75. **C. STAT CT scan head and neck without IV contrast.** A risk of a hypertensive crisis is a cerebral vascular accident (CVA). With neuro changes indicating a neurological event, a STAT head CT is the first priority to diagnose a hemorrhagic or ischemic event. rtPA would only be administered if indicated by CT scan (i.e. absense of intracranial hemorrhage). Morphine could be administered for pain, but in the big picture the patient needs to be evaluated for an acute CVA.

76. **D. ST elevation.** Acute coronary syndromes are differentiated by the presence or absence of ST elevation. Unstable angina will cause ST depression or other nonspecific changes; ST elevation indicates myocardial infarction and requires immediate treatment with percutaneous intervention or fibrinolytics. Shortness of breath and diaphoresis may be present with unstable angina. Cardiac markers will elevate in the hours following MI and can be followed to ensure that levels are falling and the infarct is resolving.

77. **C. Assess the blood glucose level.** Verify the glucose level is indeed low as the symptoms may be exhibited for other reasons. In addition, any time a patient exhibits neurologic changes, a blood glucose level should be assessed.

78. A. Antibiotics. Treatment of DIC aims to correct the underlying problem, sepsis in this case, so the appropriate intervention, would be administering antibiotics. The vital signs show no indication of shock or hemorrhage therefore administering packed red blood cells or vasoactive agents are not necessary at this time. Low dose Heparin is controversial as it may help prevent further clotting later in the DIC phase, but it may also contribute to further bleeding if administered at this time. For the most part, heparin therapy has been abandoned in DIC.

79. D. Smoking cessation and hypertension management. Age and gender are non-modifiable risk factors. Diabetes management, hypertension management and smoking cessation are all modifiable risk factors. The patient can alter his/her choice to smoke.

80. C. Pulmonary arterial hypertension. Arterial hypertension occurs from vasoconstriction of the vasculature leading to and within the lungs. Hypoxic pulmonary hypertension results from chronic low blood oxygen levels. Venous pulmonary hypertension results from left-sided heart failure and ineffective pumping of blood. Thromboembolic pulmonary hypertension results from a blood clot in the pulmonary vasculature.

81. C. Initiate a family conference with social work to discuss the issues. Since the patient is comatose, it is unclear what his wishes would be; the family's reluctance for visitors may also be multifactorial. A family conference is the appropriate setting to explore those issues with the family and determine a plan that best represents and advocates for the patient's wishes.

82. D. Request a swallow evaluation and do not administer anything by mouth. Throat clearing is an automatic failure of the bedside dysphagia screen. The patient should receive nothing by mouth and a swallow evaluation by a speech pathologist should be requested. Aspiration risk is high if the patient is allowed to have anything by mouth. Until the swallow evaluation is performed, all medications should be administered via intravenous route. If the patient does not pass the swallow evaluation, a nasogastric or enteral feeding tube may be placed for nutrition and medication administration.

83. **C. CAM assessment for delirium.** ICU & PCU patients, particularly those with longer and more complicated stays, are at risk of delirium. Evaluation of confusion in a patient with stable vitals should always include the CAM assessment.

84. **A. Symptoms of venous thrombosis.** Heparin induced thrombocytopenia (HIT) is divided into type 1, which occurs within a few days of heparin administration and resolves or stabilizes shortly thereafter, and type 2, which can cause intravascular clotting. The emboli can be limb-and life-threatening due to venous and pulmonary emboli, so immediate discontinuation of heparin and careful assessment are warranted.

85. **A. 1 L normal saline IV bolus and normal saline at 250 ml/hr.** Management of acute pancreatitis include preventing hypoxemia, resting the pancreas, pain management and supporting organ function related to inflammatory mediators. Priority multi-organ system support includes large volume fluid resuscitation due to large third spacing response to the inflammatory mediators.

86. **C. Quickly assess for a pulse.** Upon visualization of an organized rhythm during reassessment, the team must determine if the electrical activity has an associated mechanical action. A short pulse check (less than 5–10 seconds) is necessary to determine perfusion. Atropine is no longer

indicated or recommended in pulseless rhythms. Synchronized cardioversion is inappropriate as it is used to terminate tachycardic rhythms. Epinephrine is administered 1 mg every 3 to 5 minutes.

87. **C. Myocarditis.** The myocardium is the inner layer of the heart muscle, between the endocardium (inside of the heart) and pericardium (sac that surrounds the heart). Inflammation is caused by infection or injury and can occur acutely or chronically.

88. **A. Impaired renal function.** During an arteriogram, contrast dye is used to visualize the affected vessels and/or organs. Contrast dye is a nephrotoxic substance, so monitoring for impaired renal function is a priority.

89. **A. Impulsivity.** Higher cognitive functions and personality are controlled by the frontal lobe. The ability to control impulses resides in that area. Vision, language, and motor function reside in other parts of the brain.

90. **B. Uncompensated respiratory alkalosis with normal oxygen.** The pH reflects a state of alkalosis. The component that has moved in the same alkalotic direction as the pH is the $PaCO_2$. The HCO_3 has not deviated from its normal range to compensate for the disturbance. Normal oxygenation is a PaO_2 from 80–100 mm Hg on room air.

91. **B. Contact the chair of the practice council & request to add this topic to the agenda.** The practice council is the appropriate first step to determine if other staff are experiencing this as well and what resources exist within the organization to begin building a network of support.

92. **A. Tacrolimus toxicity.** Tacrolimus toxicity develops quickly as it is a medication cleared by the kidneys. Close monitoring should continue for tremors, jaundice, flushing, nephrotoxicity, and electrolyte imbalances. Medication dosing must be adjusted by the providers urgently.

93. **D. Discontinue warfarin 4–5 days prior to surgery, admission into hospital to place on IV heparin, then stop heparin 4–6 hours prior to surgery.** Interruption of anticoagulant therapy temporarily increases thromboembolic risk, and continuing anticoagulation without interruption can lead to an increase bleeding risk with invasive procedures. Stopping the long acting warfarin and allowing the INR to normalize, bridging the anticoagulant therapy using a short acting anticoagulant like heparin, will minimize the risk of perioperative thromboembolism and bleeding.

94. **A. Using a non-opioid scheduled pain protocol.** Patients with ICU & PCU stays are at high risk for developing delirium, evidenced by the agitation in this patient. Restraints and sleep medications can worsen symptoms and should be avoided. Scheduling pain medicine, frequent reorientation, providing activity during the day, and decreasing environmental stimulation are all appropriate measures. In cases of hyperactive delirium, Haldol or Seroquel could be considered. Benzodiazepines like lorazepam (Ativan) should be avoided as benzos can cause delirium and make it worse.

95. **D. Acute papillary muscle dysfunction.** The papillary muscle attaches the chordae tendineae, which control the opening and closing of the mitral valve, to the wall of the ventricle. When the muscle is damaged by a MI, the valves may become incompetent and the resulting regurgitation is audible as a murmur.

96. **B. Anastomotic leak.** Signs and symptoms of an anastomotic leak are tachycardia, tachypnea and left shoulder pain. It is possible that a MI would appear similar and collecting data to support provider decision making is important.

97. **D. Assess & documentation of a suicide risk screen.** Assessing the patient for suicide risk and documenting the findings will impact the future progression of the plan of care including minimizing restraint use, assessing for safety, and evaluating medical stability.

98. **B. Hyperglycemia, hypocalcemia, hypokalemia.** Damage to the pancreas inhibits its endocrine function of insulin production. Without insulin, hyperglycemia ensues. Lipolysis from pancreatic enzyme causes increased free fatty acids in the vascular compartment that bind calcium. Thus, the patient may exhibit hypocalcemia. Hypokalemia can result from excessive vomiting.

99. **A. Collaborate daily with the medical team to evaluate the need of the central line and urinary catheter.** Serious side effects of Depakote include an increased risk for infection, liver failure, and pancreatitis. In general, patients in the PCU should be assessed daily for discontinuation of invasive lines, tubes and drains, but this patient is at a increased risk.

100. **D. Sodium, potassium, chloride, bicarbonate.** DKA is defined as acute hyperglycemia with acidosis. It has 4 hallmark pathologies: hyperglycemia, hypovolemia, ketonemia and anion gap acidosis. The anion gap is the calculated difference between the major positively charged ions (cations), sodium and potassium, and the major negatively charged ions (anions), chloride and bicarbonate. Normal values are 0–15 mEq/L. When

the value is elevated it is indicative of an excess of unmeasurable anions in the blood and correction/resuscitation of the above pathologies must continue until the balance of cations and anions is restored. The gap is considered closed once the value normalizes.

101. D. Elevated serum osmolality. In Diabetes Insipidus there is a lack of ADH. The patient will have significant volume loss leaving an increased serum osmolality, the urine will be dilute (decreased urine osmo) and hemoconcentrated with increased sodium levels.

102. A. Beta blockers, ACE inhibitors & aldosterone antagonists. This combination of drugs reduces morbidity and mortality for patients with heart failure. Beta blockers blunt the sympathetic nervous system and lower the heart rate. ACE-inhibitors and aldosterone antagonists both help reduce preload by regulating sodium and water retention. ACE inhibitors also slow cardiac remodeling. Calcium channel blockers are typically avoided, and vasopressors are only indicated for acute exacerbations.

103. D. Cardiac tamponade. The risk of removal of epicardial pacing wires is cardiac tamponade. Clinical indications of cardiac tamponade include: hypotension, tachycardia, Pulsus paradoxus, Beck's Triad (jugular venous distension, hypotension, & muffled heart tones), altered level of consciousness, & cyanosis.

104. C. Cardiac tamponade. Cardiac tamponade is a risk after discontinuation of epicardial pacing wires. Clinical presentation of cardiac tamponade includes signs and symptoms of decreased cardiac output, increased preload and intra-cardiac pressures, and decreased contractility. In the setting of cardiac tamponade, the heart is compressed and getting "squished". All intra-cardiac pressures will increase as a result. Beck's Triad is a combination of 3 clinical signs–jugular venous distension, muffled heart sounds and hypotension.

105. **B. "We will call 911 for any signs of stroke."** The carotid artery is an important part of cerebral blood supply. Any damage or narrowing of the artery may impair cerebral blood flow and lead to an acute stroke. Patients and their families should be familiarized with the signs of stroke. A low sodium diet may be part of a plan of care, but avoiding exercise and stopping anti-hypertensives are likely not necessary.

106. **A. Position the patient with the right side down.** Following pneumonectomy, or removal of the entire lung, the operative side is placed down to allow for optimal expansion of the remaining lung. Following lobectomy, patients are positioned on the opposite side to maximize perfusion and gas exchange in the unaffected size.

107. **B. Hypokalemia.** U waves, PVCs, depressed ST segment and prolonged QT interval are all associated with hypokalemia. In hyperkalemia, peaked T waves are often observed.

108. **B. Move the patient to a bigger room and allow the ceremony to proceed as long as the environment is safe.** Advocacy for this patient means that every effort should be made to facilitate traditional customs. If it is feasible, finding a bigger space will help the group carry out their death rituals. Denying them without trying to find a solution disrespects the patient's rights.

109. **B. Contact the provider for additional orders.** Nimodipine

is a calcium channel blocker and an essential medication in the care of a patient with cerebral vasospasm and should not be held. If a patient is anticipated to be hypotensive because of the administration of this medication the providers need to be aware as they may need to begin a vasopressor or order a fluid bolus. Nimodipine is also a time sensitive medication and should be administered on time.

110. **D. Acute liver failure.** The liver is primary in gluconeogenesis and hypoglycemia or rapid decline in glucose production post-transplant may be an early sign of the new liver not functioning or experiencing acute failure or rejection.

111. **C. Dysrhythmias.** Dysrhythmias are the most common and most fatal complication of MI. Some fatal dysrhythmias may occur immediately at the time of infarct and are likely the cause of sudden death from MI, while others may develop in the next 6 months–2 years.

112. **A. Right BBB & 2nd degree Type 2 heart block.** The bundle of His and right bundle branch are located primarily in the anterior wall, so both of these may be affected in an anterior MI. 2nd degree type II heart block occurs when conduction is blocked at the bundle of His or in one of the bundle branches. If the patient develops a 2nd degree Type 2 block, you should prepare to transcutaneous pace the patient and transfer to the ICU.

113. **A. Fluid volume deficit.** The inflammatory response associated with acute pancreatitis causes increased capillary permeability and third spacing. Volume may be depleted from vomiting, diaphoresis, poor oral intake and other insensible losses. Replacing volume facilitates perfusion to organs that may suffer from coagulation and impaired fibrinolysis within

the microvasculature.

114. **C. Improve myocardial contraction.** Dobutamine is a positive inotrope that increases contractility in the heart while providing a mild reduction in afterload, both of which improve cardiac output during shock. An expected benefit of improving the cardiac output is improved urine output. However, option C is the best answer.

115. **B. Glucagon hydrochloride.** Glucagon hydrochloride is the antidote for calcium-channel antagonists and beta-adrenergic receptor antagonists. Flumazenil is given to reverse benzodiazepine effects. Naltrexone hydrochloride is given to treat alcohol or opiate dependence. Deferoxamine is used to treat acute iron toxicity.

116. **C. "Tell me more about concerns you have regarding the transfer."** The synergy model for patient care defines that nursing characteristics are derived from patient needs and must include caring practices. This includes nursing activities that create a compassionate, supportive, and therapeutic environment that promotes comfort and healing. Asking your patient to tell you about their concerns is an open-ended question that allows the patient to share their feelings without judgment. It promotes caring practices and fosters predictability for your patient.

117. **D. Immediately stop the transfusion and recheck vital signs.** Signs of a hemolytic reaction include dyspnea, chest pain, fever, chills, and acute tubular necrosis. The severity of the reaction is related to the quantity of the product received, so the transfusion should be stopped and disconnected immediately. If a reaction is suspected, samples of the transfused product

and the patient's blood are sent to the lab and/or blood bank for further testing.

118. A. Left pupil greater than right and non-reactive with noted right upper extremity extensor posturing. Assessment manifestations for cerebral insults including head bleeds and ischemic events include ipsilateral pupil changes and contralateral motor extremity changes.

119. B. Computed tomography with contrast to rule out pulmonary embolism. The patient is exhibiting signs of pulmonary embolism, which occurs more frequently in patients with pulmonary disease. CT Angio or pulmonary angiogram are the definitive tests for pulmonary embolism. Chest x-ray is nonspecific and may frequently be normal. Echocardiogram and cardiac biomarkers are not indicated for PE.

120. D. Proximal muscle weakness. Side effects of dexamethasone include decreased potassium and calcium levels, hyperglycemia, and myopathy that results in proximal muscle weakness.

121. B. Aortic stenosis. The position of the heart is such that the aorta points straight to the right sternal border, 2nd ICS. Aortic stenosis causes a systolic murmur because the narrowed valve is open during systole; a murmur of aortic insufficiency would be heard when the valve is closed during diastole.

122. D. Crackles, S$_3$ heart sound, hypotension. Left ventricular failure causes backup of blood into the pulmonary vasculature, leading to crackles, insufficient cardiac output and hypotension. The S$_3$ heart sound is caused by decreased ventricular compliance, as the ventricle is so full of blood that it is unable to stretch further.

123. **D. Abilify (aripiprazole).** Antipsychotic drugs may cause serious cardiovascular side effects including QT prolongation which may lead to Torsades de pointes and sudden cardiac death. Aripiprazole is used to treat major depression, bipolar and schizophrenia. The most common adverse effect of the drug is akathisia and has the least effect on the QT interval compared to the other medications. Seroquel, Haldol & Droperidol all have an effect on the QT interval causing prolongation.

124. **C. Maintaining a sense of self-worth.** Maintaining self-worth from age 60 until the end of life is a task of older adults. Maintaining unity with a mate, examining personal assets, and participating in organizations are tasks of middle adulthood.

125. **D. Elevated ST segment**. ST elevation is indicative of cardiac ischemia and should be treated as a myocardial infarction until proven otherwise. ECG changes associated with hyperkalemia or hypercalcemia are expected in a patient who requires dialysis.

You can do it!

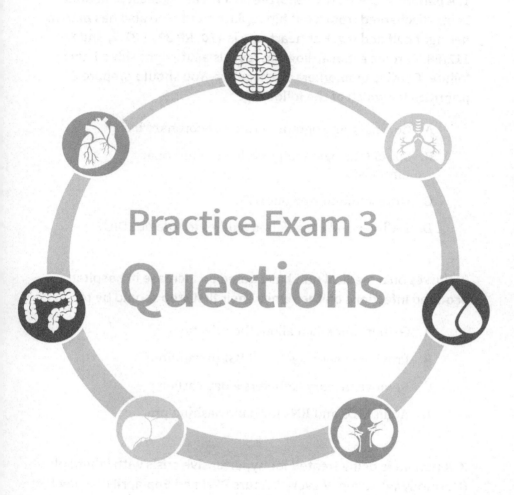

Practice Exam 3
Questions

Practice Exam #3

1. A patient presents with shortness of breath & chest pain after being discharged from a left hip replacement. She also has pain in her right calf and leg. Her heart rate is 110, RR 32, T 37.2, and BP 112/68. Cardiac echocardiogram reveals acute right sided heart failure. Cardiac biomarkers are negative. You should prepare & prioritize for which of the following?

    A. Coronary angiogram to rule out coronary lesion

    B. Spiral CT/Angio scan to rule out pulmonary embolism

    C. Ultrasound to rule out DVT

    D. D-dimer and coagulation studies to rule out DIC

2. Nurses on a medical unit have noted an increase in hospital acquired infections on their unit. Their first step should be to:

    A. Gather more data about the infections

    B. Provide in services for CLBSI prevention

    C. Remove urinary catheters a day earlier

    D. Audit MDs and RNs for handwashing practices

3. A patient is being treated for hypertensive crisis with labetalol (Normodyne) 10 mg IV every 2 hours PRN and Enalapril (Vasotec) 1.25 mg IV every 6 hours. The RN should hold the medications and notify the provider when lab findings show:

    A. ↓ Potassium

    B. ↑ Hematocrit

    C. ↓ Platelets

    D. ↑ Liver function tests

4. Which arrhythmia is commonly associated with left-sided heart failure?

    A. Atrial fibrillation

    B. 2nd degree AV block type I

    C. 2nd degree AV block type II

    D. 3rd degree AV block

5. Which set of lab values are consistent in a patient with hyperosmolar hyperglycemic non-ketotic syndrome (HHS)?

    A. Anion gap: 20; urine ketones: positive; serum potassium: 7.0; blood glucose 500 mg/dL

    B. Anion gap: 10; urine ketone: negative; serum potassium: 5.3; blood glucose 850 mg/dL

    C. Anion gap: 16; urine ketones: negative; serum potassium: 7.5; blood glucose 900 mg/dL

    D. Anion gap: 8; urine ketones: positive; serum potassium: 5.5; blood glucose 725 mg/dL

6. You are caring for a 58 year old who presented with chest discomfort and shortness of breath. A 12 Lead ECG was obtained and revealed the following:

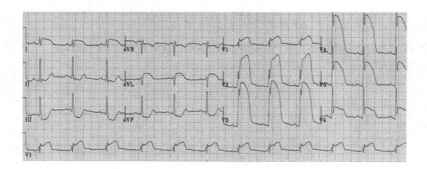

The patient had a ST-elevation myocardial infarction in which of the following walls of the heart?

   A. Antero-septal-lateral

   B. Inferior-posterior

   C. Inferior-lateral

   D. Anterior-posterior

7. Your patient just returned from an emergent CT scan of the abdomen for suspicion of acute pancreatitis. Upon arrival she is complaining of tongue swelling and difficulty breathing. You should immediately anticipate:

   A. Epinephrine 0.3 mg IM

   B. Diphenhydramine 50 mg IV

   C. Methylprednisolone 125 mg IV

   D. Epinephrine 1 mg IV

8. A murmur associated with mitral stenosis is best auscultated:

   A. At the left mid-clavicular line, during diastole

   B. At the left mid-clavicular line, during systole

   C. At the right sternal border, during diastole

   D. At the right sternal border, during systole

9. When administering Haldol to a patient with hyperactive delirium, you should closely monitor for:

   A. Reflexive tachycardia

   B. Shortened PR interval

   C. Prolonged QT interval

   D. 2nd Degree Type 1 Heart Block

10. A patient with severe vomiting may exhibit which of the following acid/base imbalances?

    A. Metabolic acidosis

    B. Metabolic alkalosis

    C. Anion gap acidosis

    D. Respiratory alkalosis

11. The nurse is caring for a patient admitted after a bicycle accident. You are told in report the patient is preparing to undergo gender reassignment surgery. What is the most appropriate statement by the nurse to establish a relationship with the patient during bedside report?

    A. "I see you are choosing to transition to the female gender"

    B. "I will call you Paul as that is what is listed on your name band"

    C. "I see the name Paul is listed on your name band, what name do you prefer to be called?"

    D. "Do you go by Paul or have you chosen your female name?"

12. A patient presents with chest pain and ST segment elevations in leads II, III and aVF. You know the patient is experiencing an infarction of which wall of the heart?

    A. Anterior wall

    B. Inferior wall

    C. Posterior wall

    D. Lateral wall

13. Torsades de Pointes is commonly associated with which of the following electrolyte disturbances?

    A. Hyperkalemia

    B. Hypokalemia

    C. Hypermagnesemia

    D. Hypomagnesemia

14. A patient with Diabetes Insipidus (DI) should be closely monitored for:

    A. Ventricular dysrhythmias

    B. S_3 ventricular gallop

    C. Hypovolemic shock

    D. Adrenal crisis

15. A 27-year-old patient has multiple open wounds and externally fixated fractures after motor vehicle collision 3 days ago. Current vitals: T 39° C, HR 106, RR 20, BP 94/60 (71). The RN notes that the patient is increasingly confused and the urine output has dropped to less than 15 ml/hour for the past 2 hours. The patient is most likely experiencing:

    A. Severe sepsis

    B. Bacteremia

    C. SIRS

    D. Sepsis

16. A patient with chronic, severe mitral insufficiency is prone to which of the following dysrhythmias?

    A. Complete heart block

    B. AV Dissociation

    C. Atrial fibrillation

    D. Second degree AV Block, Type I

17. A medication regimen for a patient with hypertrophic cardiomyopathy may include:

    A. Cardiac glycosides & beta blockers

    B. Beta blockers & vasopressors

    C. Calcium channel blockers & beta blockers

    D. Vasopressors & Inotropes

18. You are caring for a patient with diabetes who has a history of arterial insufficiency and peripheral neuropathy. You note a wound under their heel that is even, well-defined and has variable amounts of exudate. Which of the following wounds do you suspect your patient most likely to have?

    A. Arterial ulcer

    B. Venous ulcer

    C. Pressure ulcer

    D. Diabetic ulcer

19. The nurse is caring for a 70-year-old female patient admitted for sepsis. At 20:00 the patient is noted to have an acute fluctuation in mental status, is restless and demonstrating inattention. The nurse determines she is CAM positive for delirium. Which intervention by the nurse is the most appropriate next step?

    A. Administer an intravenous anxiolytic

    B. Collaborate with the medical provider to determine the appropriate level of restraint and sedation therapy

    C. Discuss the confusion with her family, ensuring them it is normal

    D. Collaborate with the provider to minimize delirium inducing medications and develop a plan to facilitate sleep

20. Post-Traumatic Stress Disorder (PTSD) includes which of the following?

    A. A mental health disorder that is triggered by a terrifying event

    B. A mental health disorder with symptoms similar to hyperactivity

    C. A mental health disorder that does not respond to psychotherapy

    D. A mental health disorder that accompanies all critical illness

21. A 68-year-old patient with COPD presents with SOB. He is given a nebulizer treatment, but remains SOB. An ABG reveals the following: pH 7.32/PaCO$_2$ 54/ PaO$_2$ 103/ HCO$_3$ 28.

This ABG confirms:

A. Uncompensated metabolic acidosis

B. Partially compensated metabolic alkalosis

C. Partially compensated respiratory acidosis

D. Compensated respiratory alkalosis

22. A patient is admitted to the hospital with abdominal pain and nausea and was taken to the operating room for an emergent bowel resection. The post-operative course has been complicated by septic shock and acute kidney injury (AKI). The patient is placed on intermittent hemodialysis. The nurse recognizes which of the following is a priority to ensure safe patient care while receiving renal replacement therapy?

A. Invasive hemodynamic monitoring to assess fluid volume status hourly

B. Frequent electrolyte monitoring to identify electrolyte shifts

C. Hourly urine output monitoring to know when hemodialysis should be discontinued

D. Daily weight monitoring to assess fluid status

23. A patient with end-stage heart failure is becoming more depressed and withdrawn. You feel music therapy may help. What steps should you take prior to instituting music therapy?

    A. Ask the patient if he likes music & what type

    B. Get a provider's order

    C. Ensure all nursing tasks have been completed

    D. Consult the psychiatry team because he is depressed

24. A 52-year-old male just underwent a 3 vessel CABG. He has been in NSR and suddenly converts to atrial fibrillation at a rate of 160. His BP suddenly drops to 72/46 (54) & is feeling short of breath. You should anticipate which of the following?

    A. Adenosine 6 mg rapid IVP

    B. Defibrillation with 100 joules

    C. Synchronized cardioversion with 100 joules

    D. Diltiazem bolus followed by an infusion

25. Which of the following is an example of advocacy?

    A. Standing behind organizational decisions that are formed based on the needs of patients

    B. Working with individuals to create synergistic relationships

    C. Consistently acting with intention and upholding ethical values and principles

    D. Being an honest and trustworthy individual

26. A right sided tension pneumothorax is suspected in your patient who acutely dropped her oxygen saturation to 82%. Physical signs may include:

  A. Tracheal deviation to the left and absent breath sounds over the pneumothorax

  B. Tracheal deviation to the right and absent breath sounds over the pneumothorax

  C. Tracheal deviation to the left and adventitious breath sounds over the pneumothorax

  D. Tracheal deviation to the right and adventitious breath sounds over the pneumothorax

27. A 78-year-old female experienced a fall at home 1 week ago. She has been on Coumadin for atrial fibrillation for over 1 year. She presents with a complaint of headache. Her family states: "Mom has been acting weird for the past couple of days." This scenario is consistent with:

  A. Arteriovenous malformation rupture

  B. Cerebral aneurysm rupture

  C. Epidural hematoma

  D. Subdural hematoma

28. The Confusion Assessment Method scale (CAM) is useful in identifying which of the following acute disorders:

  A. Post-traumatic Stress Disorder

  B. Dementia

  C. Delirium

  D. Depression

29. During a patient's admission to the PCU, the RN notes a hemoglobin level of 9 g/dL and hematocrit of 27 mL/dL. Which medication should be confirmed with the provider prior to administration?

    A. Metoprolol (Toprol)

    B. Sulfa-trimethoprim (Bactrim)

    C. Erythropoietin (EPO)

    D. Furosemide (Lasix)

30. A 73-year-old female is in the PCU for acute coronary syndrome. She is complaining of dizziness, chest pain, and nausea. You look up at the bedside monitor and see the following rhythm:

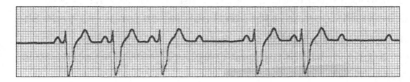

You interpret the rhythm as:

    A. 1st degree AV block

    B. 2nd degree AV block type I

    C. 2nd degree AV block type II

    D. 3rd degree AV block

31. Which leads on a 12 Lead ECG would you assess for changes associated with an anterior wall myocardial infarction?

    A. I, aVL, V_5, V_6

    B. II, III, aVF

    C. V_1 & V_2

    D. V_3 & V_4

32. A 56-year-old male presents in heart block with a ventricular rate of 38 caused from an intentional overdose from calcium channel blockers. What is the appropriate antidote?

    A. Glucagon

    B. Diphenhydramine

    C. Calcium

    D. Atropine

33. Your patient was admitted due to severe dehydration in the setting of chronic alcoholism. The patient is complaining of severe "stabbing" abdominal pain that radiates to their back. The skin is mottled. Which of the following labs and diet do you expect the provider to order?

    A. Lipase & amylase, NPO and a bolus of IV fluids

    B. ALT & AST, clear liquid diet and increase oral fluids

    C. Complete metabolic panel, troponin and cardiac prudent diet

    D. BUN & creatinine and NPO status

34. A patient on the intermediate care unit is post-operative day 2 after a right hemicolectomy for ischemic bowel. The post-operative course has been complicated with pain control concerns. As the patient is getting out of bed for the first time, the patient complains of sudden onset shortness of breath and anxiety with a sudden wet sounding cough. The nurse assesses new onset tachycardia with a wide complex QRS. The nurse suspects which complication?

    A. Anterior wall MI

    B. Pulmonary embolism

    C. Tension pneumothorax

D. Anastomosis rupture

35. You are caring for a patient who does not speak English. What is the best way to communicate with the patient?

    A. Ask the family member that does speak English to translate

    B. Use a certified translation service

    C. Use a translation mobile application

    D. Ask the patient closed-ended questions to elicit a "yes" or "no" response

36. Which of the following lab profiles would you expect to see in a patient with acute pancreatitis?

    A. Elevated amylase, lipase & albumin

    B. Elevated albumin, decreased amylase & lipase

    C. Decreased albumin, elevated amylase & lipase

    D. Decreased albumin, amylase & lipase

37. A 65-year-old patient has been in the PCU for 3 days with acute decompensated left ventricular heart failure. The patient's heart rate is 78, BP 94/64 with urine output averaging 50 ml/hr. On assessment, you note a S3 heart sound and crackles through the mid lung fields. What should you anticipate next?

    A. Continuous monitoring as the measurement is normal

    B. Dobutamine infusion at 5 mcg/kg/min

    C. Furosemide 20 mg IV x 1

    D. 500 ml lactated ringers bolus x 1

38. A patient presents with an anterior wall MI and goes into a 2nd degree Type II heart bock at a rate of 36 bpm. The BP is 72/46 (54). What is the next appropriate intervention?

   A. Call for help and prepare to transcutaneous pace

   B. Call for help and administer atropine 0.5 mg IV

   C. Call for help and prepare for defibrillation

   D. Notify the provider

39. You are caring for a patient who inadvertently took too many warfarin tablets. His INR is 6.2 and he has blood in his stool. His hematocrit has dropped from 39 to 30. Which of the following is most effective in reversing the warfarin?

   A. Protamine

   B. Cryoprecipitate

   C. Platelets

   D. Vitamin K

40. You are caring for a patient admitted with Hyperosmolar Hyperglycemic Non-ketotic Syndrome (HHS) and a new diagnosis of Diabetes Mellitus Type II. The patient will likely be discharged within the next 24–48 hours. In providing education for the patient, you should first:

   A. Educate the patient about everything they need to know about diabetes

   B. Provide a handout that explains diabetes

   C. Ask the patient what they already know about diabetes

   D. Have the patient inject their insulin themselves to prepare them for home injections.

41. A patient with a new diagnosis of Stage 4 pancreatic cancer is admitted to your unit. A palliative care consult has been requested by the admitting medical providers. The nurse informs the patient of the planned consult. The patient states "Just because I have cancer, I have to go on hospice? I thought I had the right to try treatment?" The best response by the nurse is:

    A. "I will call the doctor and cancel the consult"

    B. "Palliative care is something we do this for every patient diagnosed with your type of cancer. You still make decisions"

    C. "Hospice and palliative care are different. I can get someone to talk to you about it"

    D. "Palliative care is a great resource to support your goals for treatment and quality of life as you make decisions about your care"

42. When caring for a patient with a traumatic brain injury, which intervention should you include to help prevent an increase in intracranial pressure?

    A. Keep the patient's head in a neutral midline position

    B. Keep the head of bed flat at all times

    C. Keep the patient slightly hyperthermic

    D. Administer oxygen to keep the patient slightly hyperoxemic

43. You are caring for a patient with an acute episode of asthma exacerbation. The first line of treatment is:

A. Corticosteroids

B. Beta$_2$ agonist

C. IV fluids

D. Chest x-ray to rule out pneumonia

44. A 46-year-old patient presents with pneumonia and sepsis. He was treated with 4 days of antibiotics and IV fluids. He is increasingly short of breath and is now on 100% O_2 via non-re-breather mask. A Rapid Response is activated.

You obtain an ABG with the following results: pH 7.20 / $PaCO_2$ 68/ PaO_2 102/ HCO_3 28. A chest x-ray reveals bilateral pulmonary infiltrates. The patient is likely developing:

A. Worsening pneumonia

B. Acute Respiratory Distress Syndrome

C. Pulmonary embolus

D. Atelectasis

45. You are caring for a patient with a serum potassium level of 3.0. The admission potassium was 4.2. Which of the following is the most likely cause of the sudden drop in potassium?

A. Dehydration from diarrhea

B. Loop diuretics

C. Acidosis

D. Blood transfusion

46. A 78-year-old female patient is experiencing hyperactive delirium. She is trying to pull out her bladder catheter and get out of bed. What is the medication of choice to treat hyperactive delirium?

    A. Diazepam

    B. Haloperidol

    C. Lorazepam

    D. Midazolam

47. Which assessment score should be completed within one hour of presentation of stroke, evaluates the severity of ischemic stroke and is a predictor of patient outcome?

    A. Hunt & Hess Scale

    B. Miami Emergency Neurologic Deficit Scale (MEND)

    C. National Institute of Health Stroke Scale (NIHSS)

    D. Cincinnati Pre-hospital Stroke Scale (CPSS)

48. Acetylsalicylic acid (aspirin) is a non-steroidal anti-inflammatory medication that inhibits the release of which of the following?

    A. Platelets

    B. Fibrinogen

    C. Thromboxane A_2

    D. Nitric Oxide

49. Bone marrow transplant failure with leukemia can present with clinical manifestations of which of the following?

    A. Decreased risk of infection and anemia

    B. Increased risk of infection and hypercoagulation

    C. Increased risk of infection, bleeding and anemia

    D. Hypercoagulation and anemia

50. The benefit of the Trans-jugular intrahepatic portosystemic shunt (TIPS) procedure is:

    A. Stop esophageal bleeding

    B. Relieve portal venous pressure

    C. Prevent liver enzyme elevation

    D. Increase blood flow to the liver

51. Which type of the following heart block complications would you monitor for in the setting of an anterior wall MI?

    A. 1st degree AV block

    B. 2nd degree Type I (Wenckebach)

    C. 2nd degree Type II

    D. Sinus bradycardia

52. Which of the following is a complication of infective endocarditis?

    A. Myocarditis

    B. Heart failure

    C. Emboli

    D. Pericarditis

53. A patient with severe GERD admitted with aspiration pneumonia is prescribed IV ampicillin. Ampicillin is transitioned to an oral tablet as the patient's condition improves. The nurse understands the importance of higher gastric pH to ensure the effectiveness of ampicillin in treatment. Which is the appropriate next step for the nurse?

A. Review prescribed medications with the provider in daily rounds

B. Contact the pharmacist to prevent concomitant administration of both medications

C. Provide patient education regarding increasing dietary acid

D. Administer the medications as prescribed

54. You are caring for a 55 year old patient who experienced an acute anterior wall myocardial infarction and developed acute tubular necrosis (ATN). The patient has been anuric for 2 days and is currently receiving intermittent dialysis with an order to perform ultrafiltration only. Because of this, you know the goal of the therapy is to:

A. Remove cytokines

B. Remove fluid only

C. Rapid removal of excess electrolytes, such as potassium

D. Remove metabolic waste such as urea nitrogen and creatinine

55. A 54-year-old patient with no significant medical history is admitted to the PCU 3 days following elective clipping of a cerebral aneurysm. Which of the following assessment findings is most concerning?

    A. Subjective complaint of a 6/10 headache

    B. Drowsiness

    C. Left-sided pronator drift

    D. Inability to remember the date

56. The purpose of mediastinal chest tubes in a patient post-operative Day 2 from a 3 vessel CABG is to:

    A. Drain serosanguinous drainage post-op

    B. Improve alveolar expansion

    C. Re-expand the lungs

    D. Remove blood from the pleural space

57. What is the most important nursing goal in caring for the patient with Hepatitis C?

    A. Adequate nutrition

    B. Maintenance of skin integrity

    C. Prevention of the spread of the virus

    D. Promotion of positive body image

58. Which of the following is used to treat coronary vasospasm caused by variant angina?

    A. An alpha-adrenergic blocking agent

    B. A beta-adrenergic blocking agent

    C. A calcium channel-blocking agent

    D. A cholinergic agent

59. You are conducting the admission health history on a 56-year-old female patient diagnosed with an acute antero-septal wall MI. You ask the patient if she has an advanced directive or living will and she does not respond. You next hear an alarm at the bedside monitor. The patient is unresponsive and you see the following rhythm on the monitor:

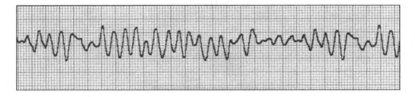

What is your next action?

    A. Call for help and immediately start CPR

    B. Call for help and administer Magnesium 1 gm IV

    C. Call for help and prepare for synchronized cardioversion

    D. Call for help and administer Amiodarone 300 mg IV

60. Signs of a small bowel infarction include:

   A. Diarrhea & increased bilirubin

   B. Hypoactive bowel sounds & leukocytosis

   C. Tympanic sounds over the abdomen

   D. Hyperactive bowel sounds & jaundice

61. A 24-year-old male patient is admitted with a large stab wound to the abdomen and exploratory laparotomy. Two days post-op, the patient has the following vital signs: T 38.6° C, P 114, R 24, BP 90/72. WBC: 18,500. Upon notifying the provider, what should the nurse anticipate next?

   A. Administration of acetaminophen and a broad spectrum IV antibiotic

   B. Preparation for emergency surgery

   C. STAT abdominal x-ray

   D. STAT serum lactate and blood cultures

62. A 36-year-old female patient is admitted to the PCU status-post motor vehicle collision. She was an unrestrained passenger. The patient is observed to have bruising around the eyes and behind the ears. Which of the following nursing diagnoses has the highest priority given this information?

   A. Fluid volume deficit

   B. Ineffective airway clearance

   C. Potential for infection

   D. Potential for skin breakdown

63. A patient with pneumonia has been sustaining a respiratory rate of 25–30 per minute and SpO$_2$ 93% on a 60% facemask. The nurse should activate the Rapid Response Team and notify the provider for immediate intubation when they observe:

    A. Nostril flaring

    B. RR 20 with shallow breathing and decreased LOC

    C. Increased accessory muscle use

    D. SaO$_2$ 91%

64. A 61-year-old female is admitted with fluid overload in the setting of chronic kidney disease. Her serum calcium level is 13.5 mg/dL. Which sign is this patient likely to exhibit?

    A. Shortened QT interval on the ECG

    B. Trousseau sign

    C. Grey-Turner's sign

    D. Positive Chvostek sign

65. The family of a 79-year-old female was just told she passed away after unsuccessful cardiac resuscitation. They view her body and are crying. Your best immediate action would be:

    A. Provide a private quiet room so they can spend time alone

    B. Ask them if they would like you to call the medical examiner

    C. Ask if they would like her wedding rings removed

    D. Provide names of some good funeral homes

66. A patient with an inferior wall MI and right ventricular infarction develops tachycardia and hypotension. What would be the best initial treatment for hypotension?

    A. Nitroglycerin infusion

    B. Dopamine infusion

    C. Dobutamine infusion

    D. Normal saline boluses

67. You are caring for a 62 year old male admitted with chest pain, rule out myocardial infarction. His initial troponins were slightly elevated and a cardiac catheterization is planned. While assessing his morning ECG rhythm strip, you notice his corrected QT interval is 0.46 seconds. Which of the following medications should you be concerned about administering?

    A. Ondansetron

    B. Lisinopril

    C. Paroxetine

    D. Potassium

68. Which of the following is the highest priority when providing discharge education with a patient who is a Type II Diabetic s/p Gastric Bypass surgery?

    A. Notify your provider if you have leg cramping

    B. Notify your provider if you only lose 5 pounds

    C. Watch for signs of hypoglycemia

    D. Watch for signs of low platelets

69. A new pressure ulcer prevention dressing has been purchased and a protocol developed for placement on the coccyx of patients on bedrest. The nurse is caring for the second spinal cord injury patient with a rapidly developed deep tissue injury on their coccyx. Which is the appropriate next step by the nurse?

    A. Stop using the product and take them off

    B. File a safety report recording the lack of assessment by the previous nurse

    C. File a safety report and bring it to the attention of nursing leadership

    D. Talk with your coworkers about your findings

70. You suspect your patient is developing cardiac tamponade after epicardial pacing wire removal. Which of the following are clinical manifestations you may notice in the setting of cardiac tamponade?

    A. Normal heart sounds, bradycardia with hypertension & normal jugular vein

    B. Muffled heart sounds, tachycardia with hypotension & jugular vein distention

    C. S_3, tachycardia, narrowing pulse pressure with hypertension & a murmur

    D. Positive Pulsus Paradoxes, bradycardia & wide pulse pressure

71. A severely depressed diabetic patient is admitted after taking a large amount of insulin in an attempt to commit suicide. Asking about suicidal thoughts and feelings will help you ascertain:

    A. If they have a specific plan to attempt suicide again

    B. Place the patient on suicide watch

    C. Give them ideas for successful suicide

    D. If they are more depressed

72. Common clinical manifestations of cardiogenic shock include:

    A. Decreased afterload

    B. Decreased preload

    C. Expiratory wheezes

    D. Cool, pale, moist skin

73. You are caring for a patient who developed septic shock due to pneumonia and a blood stream infection. You are concerned that the patient may be showing signs of Disseminated Intravascular Coagulation (DIC). Which of the following would you expect to see in a patient with DIC?

    A. Purpura and petechiae

    B. Decreased PT & PTT

    C. Elevated platelet count

    D. Spider angiomas

74. The most important factor when determining a plan for mobility for a patient recovering from septic shock is:

    A. Optimization of oxygenation

    B. Presence of a nasogastric or other enteral feeding tube

    C. The number of intravenous medication infusions

    D. The patient's ability to be alert and follow commands

75. The nurse is caring for a patient with tachypnea, dyspnea at rest, hemoptysis, and JVD. The patient returned from the Cath lab after a right heart catheterization. The patient was diagnosed with Pulmonary Arterial Hypertension. The right heart cath findings likely included:

    A. Decreased right heart preload

    B. Normal left heart preload

    C. Decreased pulmonary vascular resistance

    D. Elevated pulmonary artery pressure

76. Which lab value would the nurse expect to find in a patient with venous thromboembolism?

    A. aPTT 50 seconds

    B. D-dimer 650 ng/mL

    C. Platelet 100 thousand/mm^3

    D. Fibrinogen 220 mg/dL

77. A patient admitted to the hospital with severe vomiting for two days after beginning chemotherapy. The nurse notices a sudden change in the color of the emesis to bright red. What complication does the nurse suspect?

    A. Esophageal variceal rupture

    B. Gastric perforation

    C. Gastritis

    D. Mallory-Weiss Tear

78. A patient recently admitted with congestive heart failure is being treated with loop diuretics. What signs of hypokalemia would be evident on the ECG?

    A. Tachycardia

    B. Peaked T waves

    C. U waves

    D. Widened QRS

79. A patient presents in heart failure with acute shortness of breath. When auscultating lung sounds you observe crackles through all the lung fields. You also expect to hear which heart tone?

    A. S_4

    B. Split S_1

    C. Pericardial friction rub

    D. S_3

80. Which of the following is initially indicated for blunt cardiac trauma in the setting of hypoperfusion and hypotension?

A. Inotropes

B. Afterload reducers

C. IV fluids

D. Intra-aortic balloon counterpulsation

81. A patient is receiving haloperidol (Haldol) for delirium. The RN notes new onset of tremors and slurred speech. The best response is to:

A. Administer diphenhydramine (Benadryl) 25 mg IV push

B. Administer anti-seizure medication early

C. Call the stroke team STAT

D. Administer Romazicon (Flumazenil) 0.2 mg IV push

82. A patient with a history of seizures was admitted for pneumonia several days ago. As the nurse completes an assessment, the patient begins to experience a generalized tonic-clonic seizure, which persists for several minutes. The best initial intervention is to:

A. Administer the prescribed antiepileptic drug

B. Call a code and prepare to intubate

C. Place an oral airway and administer oxygen

D. Turn the patient to their side and set up suction equipment

83. You are caring for a 42-year-old female with chronic right-sided heart failure. Her vital signs are: HR 102 in atrial fibrillation, BP: 102/72 (82), respirations: 20/minute, SpO$_2$: 95% on 4 liters per nasal cannula. What should you expect to find during your physical assessment in the setting of right sided heart failure?

    A. Bibasilar crackles throughout the lung fields

    B. Decreased urine output

    C. Hepato-Jugular reflex sign

    D. Opacities on the chest radiograph

84. A patient with chronic pulmonary arterial hypertension is admitted to the unit. The nurse reconciles the home medication list and expects it to include:

    A. Metoprolol, furosemide, and aspirin

    B. Diphenhydramine, warfarin, and diltiazem

    C. Aspirin, atenolol, and metformin

    D. Warfarin, furosemide, and amlodipine

85. The nurse is caring for a patient who speaks Farsi and has a bilingual family member at the bedside. It is most appropriate to allow the family to translate when:

    A. Determining code status

    B. Assessing comfort

    C. Signing consent

    D. Planning transfer to skilled nursing facility

86. Which of the following assessment findings would you expect to find in septic shock?

    A. Bradycardia, Hypertension, Hypothermia

    B. Bradycardia, Hypotension, Hyperthermia

    C. Tachycardia, Hypertension, Hypothermia

    D. Tachycardia, Hypotension, Hyperthermia

87. The Rapid Response Team is activated for a patient on hospital day 2 admitted after an anterior wall myocardial infarction (MI). The patient is anxious, pale, and dyspneic with tachypnea. The patient has had minimal urine output the past 4 hours. Vital signs are as follows:

    HR 128

    BP 92/46(61)

    RR 38

The provider orders for the patient to be transferred to the ICU, but the bed is not available.

Which of the following medication regimens should the nurse anticipate to treat cardiogenic shock to improve cardiac output?

    A. Esmolol (Brevibloc) 50 mcg/kg/min and 1 Liter normal saline bolus

    B. Norepinephrine 0.02 mcg/kg/min and 40 mg IV Furosemide (Lasix) 40 mg IV

    C. Furosemide (Lasix) 40 mg IV and a Dobutamine infusion at 2.5 mcg/kg/min

    D. 1 Liter normal saline bolus and a Dobutamine infusion at 5 mcg/kg/min

88. You are caring for a 54-year-old patient with acute pancreatitis. What is the proper order to perform an abdominal examination?

A. Percussion, auscultation, palpation

B. Palpation, inspection, auscultation

C. Auscultation, inspection, palpation

D. Inspection, auscultation, palpation

89. Which of the following signs compose "Cushing's Triad" in the setting of cerebral herniation?

A. Tachycardia, systolic hypertension, narrow pulse pressure

B. Bradycardia, diastolic hypertension, wide pulse pressure

C. Tachycardia, diastolic hypertension, narrow pulse pressure

D. Bradycardia, systolic hypertension, wide pulse pressure

90. A 68-year-old female inadvertently overdosed on her beta blocker medication. On admission her VS are: HR 38, BP 72/38 (46), RR 22, O_2 sat 94%. The ECG monitor is showing 2nd degree block Type 2. What is your immediate priority for this patient?

A. Administer 1 amp of Calcium Chloride IV

B. Administer Glucagon 3 mg IV

C. Administer Atropine 0.5 mg IV

D. Administer Dextrose 50 1 amp IV

91. What does the Glasgow coma scale assess?

    A. Motor response, eye opening, hearing

    B. Eye opening, sensory response, motor response

    C. Sensory response, verbal response, motor response

    D. Motor response, verbal response, eye opening

92. A patient required 4 units of PRBCs for GI Bleeding. Which of the following electrolytes do you anticipate replacing?

    A. Calcium

    B. Magnesium

    C. Phosphate

    D. Potassium

93. In the care of a patient with diabetic ketoacidosis the nurse understands that end goals of treatment include:

    A. Widening of the anion gap, maintaining serum K^+ above 3.3 mEq/L, and normalization of the blood glucose below 250 mg/dl

    B. Closure of the anion gap, maintaining serum K^+ above 3.3 mEq/L, and decreasing the blood glucose below 250 mg/dl

    C. Closure of the cation gap, elevation of the serum bicarbonate, and normalization of the blood glucose below 150 mg/dl.

    D. Closure of the anion gap, increase in the serum osmolality, and elevation of the serum bicarbonate level

94. The provider orders a 3% saline infusion @ 30 ml/hour for a patient with severe hyponatremia. What should the nurse consider regarding administration of this IV fluid?

   A. IV administration requires the use of a central venous catheter

   B. Sodium replacement should not exceed 0.5 mEq/L per hour

   C. Total daily replacement should not exceed 18 mEq/L

   D. Notify the physician once the serum sodium is 145 mEq/L

95. A patient presents to your unit with a bleeding gastric ulcer. Which pathogen is most commonly associated with causing gastric ulcers?

   A. Helicobacter pylori

   B. Escherichia coli

   C. Staphylococcus aureus

   D. Clostridium difficile

96. You are caring for a 62-year-old patient with advanced cirrhosis and end stage liver disease. He is having difficulty breathing from his ascites. VS: HR 102, RR 30, BP 102/56 (62), O2 sat 92%. Which of the following would be most beneficial?

   A. Administer albumin

   B. Administer lactulose

   C. Place in reverse Trendelenburg & administer furosemide

   D. Place on 100% NRB mask

97. Your patient has a closed head injury and becomes febrile with a temperature of 39.9° C. The critical care nurse understands that an increase in temperature:

A. Is easily lowered with acetaminophen

B. Improves intracranial pressure

C. Increases oxygen requirements of the brain tissue

D. Offers no threat to the neurological system

98. A patient with a partial intestinal obstruction caused by abdominal adhesions may find relief with which of the following diets?

A. High fiber, low protein

B. High fiber, high dairy

C. Low fiber, low dairy

D. Low fiber, high protein

99. You are caring for an 18 year-old patient Type I diabetic that presented with Diabetic Ketoacidosis (DKA). You know that they are in the initial phase of DKA from which of the following lab findings?

A. Hyperphosphatemia & hyperglycemia

B. Hyperphosphatemia & metabolic acidosis

C. Decreased plasma osmolality & ketones in the urine

D. Hyperkalemia & hyponatremia

100. You are admitting a patient s/p elective clipping of a cerebral aneurysm. Which of the following nursing actions should you anticipate?

    A. Administer Mannitol every 12 hours to reduce cerebral edema

    B. Position with the head of bed 30 degrees to optimize venous outflow

    C. Decrease the MAP to improve the CPP

    D. Monitor for delirium

101. Interpret the following arterial blood gases:

    pH 7.29 / PaCO$_2$ 38 / PaO$_2$ 65 / HCO$_3$ 18

    A. Partially compensated respiratory acidosis with mild hypoxia

    B. Partially compensated metabolic acidosis with moderated hypoxia

    C. Uncompensated respiratory acidosis with moderate hypoxia

    D. Uncompensated metabolic acidosis with mild hypoxia

102. A staff RN receives report on a new admission and feels the acuity is too high with her current assignment. The charge nurse's best response is to:

    A. Reassign the admission to another nurse

    B. Reassign the RN's current patients to another nurse

    C. Discuss assignments with the nurses involved

    D. Ask the staffing office for an additional RN

103. A 31-year-old male was admitted to the PCU with bradycardia, hypotension and altered mental status. Which of the following substances could likely be the cause of this symptomology?

    A. Aspirin

    B. Phenobarbital

    C. Alcohol

    D. Cocaine

104. Which of the following class of medications should be avoided in cocaine induced myocardial infarctions?

    A. Calcium channel blockers

    B. ACE Inhibitors

    C. Aldosterone antagonists

    D. Beta blockers

105. You are caring for a 43 year old female who presents with chest pain. She had a myocardial infarction 2 weeks ago. She states her pain is better when she sits up and leans forward. She has taken 3 sublingual Nitroglycerin tablets with no relief. Ibuprofen is the only medication that seems to decrease her pain. Upon physical examination, you note a pericardial friction rub.

Here is her 12 Lead ECG:

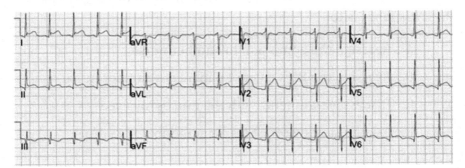

You suspect which of the following?

   A. Acute pericarditis

   B. Acute anterior wall myocardial infarction

   C. Acute papillary muscle rupture

   D. Acute inferior wall myocardial infarction

106. A 47-year-old patient is admitted following ingestion of an undetermined amount of salicylates approximately 4 hours ago. After initial stabilization in the Emergency Department the patient is acidotic but stable. The treatment priority to correct the acidosis should include which of the following?

   A. Sodium bicarbonate

   B. Hemodialysis

   C. Activated charcoal

   D. N-acetylcysteine

107. Calcium is necessary in producing a blood clot by which of the following mechanisms?

   A. Calcium binds with fibrinogen

   B. Forming clots when calcium reacts with Factor Xa

   C. Calcium is the by-product of the thyroid gland

   D. Calcium being released from the parathyroid gland

108. A patient on Dilantin for a seizure disorder presents with dilutional hyponatremia after a recent respiratory infection. The current sodium level is 124. Which of the following is likely the cause of the electrolyte derangement?

    A. Elevated TSH

    B. Elevated T3 & T4

    C. Excessive ADH

    D. Parathyroid dysfunction

109. A patient presents to your unit complaining of nausea, diaphoresis and chest heaviness. A repeat 12 Lead ECG is performed and reveals the following:

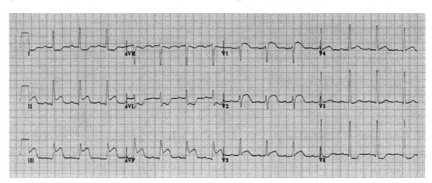

Based on these findings, you suspect the patient has an occlusion in which of the following arteries?

    A. Left anterior descending artery

    B. Proximal artery

    C. Left main artery

    D. Right coronary artery

110. Which of the following laboratory findings should be expected in a patient with acute pancreatitis?

    A. Hypercalcemia & hypokalemia

    B. Hypocalcemia & hyperglycemia

    C. Hyperkalemia & Hypocalcemia

    D. Hyperglycemia & Hypercalcemia

111. You are performing a cardiovascular assessment and want to auscultate the pulmonic valve. Where would you place your stethoscope?

    A. 2nd ICS; right sternal border

    B. 2nd ICS; left sternal border

    C. 3rd ICS; left sternal border

    D. 5th ICS; midclavicular line

112. A patient hospitalized for septic pneumonia has developed hematemesis with a suspected bleeding gastric ulcer. The collaborative plan has been developed to include endoscopic evaluation the following morning. Which pharmacological intervention is a priority in the care of this client?

    A. Octreotide 25 mcg/hr IV infusion

    B. Pantoprazole 8 mg/hr IV infusion

    C. Ranitidine 150 mg IV every 8 hours

    D. Ondansetron 4 mg IV every 8 hours

113. You are transporting a 50-year-old female to the radiology department for a MRI of the brain. After the contrast dye is injected, the patient states: "I'm not feeling too well. My tongue feels thick and my throat is scratchy." What should you anticipate doing next?

A. Call for help, support airway/breathing, prepare to give diphenhydramine 50 mg IV

B. Call for help, support airway/breathing, prepare to give Epinephrine (1:1000) 0.3 mg IM

C. Call for help, support airway/breathing, prepare to give Epinephrine (1:10,000) 0.5 mg IV

D. Call for help, support airway/breathing, prepare to give Epinephrine (1:1000) 1 mg IV

114. You are caring for a patient with an exacerbation of Chronic Obstructive Pulmonary Disease (COPD). The patient is placed on non-invasive ventilation (Bi-Pap) for suspected hypercapnia. An arterial blood gas is obtained with the following result:

pH 7.30

$PaCO_2$ 68

PaO_2 94

HCO_3 34

SaO_2 93%

How would you interpret the arterial blood gas?

A. Uncompensated metabolic acidosis

B. Partially compensated respiratory acidosis

C. Uncompensated respiratory alkalosis

D. Partially compensated metabolic alkalosis

115. The nurse is caring for a patient being treated for resolving septic shock over the past 5 days. The patient required large volume fluid resuscitation and was extubated 2 days ago. The nurse assesses the patient and notes increased work of breathing and jugular venous distension (JVD) with circumoral cyanosis. The patient is extremely anxious. Patient data is as follows:

HR 140

BP 68/42 (50)

RR 32

O_2 saturation is 85% on 80% FiO_2

Which pharmacological intervention does the nurse anticipate to treat the highly suspected pulmonary embolism?

A. Alteplase (Activase) 100 mg IV over 2 hours

B. Norepinephrine 0.3 mcg/kg/min

C. Heparin 5000 units SubQ injection every 12 hours

D. Warfarin 5 mg per feeding tube q HS

116. A patient with chronic renal failure presents with a history of nausea/vomiting, diarrhea, tingling skin, and confusion. A 12-lead ECG shows tall tented T waves with a widened QRS, prolonged PR interval and wide P waves. These findings are consistent with which of the following electrolyte disturbances?

A. Hypomagnesemia

B. Hypermagnesemia

C. Hypokalemia

D. Hyperkalemia

117. In review of monthly hospital readmission data the nurse recognizes an upward trend in readmission rates for patients with heart failure. Which action by the nurse demonstrates an understanding of the impact of patient education on hospital readmission rates?

    A. Convene inter-professional team to review missing required patient education and establish standard processes for documentation of discharge education

    B. Collaborate with the clinical practice education department to create learning module for all nurses complete regarding required patient education

    C. Collaborate with nursing education department to create a patient education lecture for new hire nurse orientation

    D. Work with the nurse manager to complete audits of the inter-professional education record and provide feedback to staff documenting discharge education

118. You are caring for a 32 year old admitted with septic shock. She has been hospitalized for 5 days and now is oozing blood from mucous membranes, has multiple bruises and guaiac positive stool. Her labs reveal the following: Hct 29, platelet count 12,000, fibrinogen 96, PT 14, INR 2.2, aPTT 38. DIC is suspected. Which of the following do you anticipate?

    A. Transfusion of PRBCs

    B. Start heparin infusion

    C. Transfusion of platelets & cryoprecipitate

    D. Administration of vitamin K

119. Which of the following patients is highest risk for developing diabetes insipidus?

    A. 18-year-old traumatic brain injury

    B. 65-year-old Type II diabetic

    C. 89-year-old with delirium

    D. 48-year-old with sepsis

120. A 56-year-old female presents with sub-sternal chest pain radiating to her left arm and jaw. After initial assessment, a 12-lead ECG is performed and reveals ST segment elevation in leads II, III, & aVF. You would expect reciprocal changes in which leads?

    A. V_1, V_2

    B. I, aVL

    C. aVR, aVL, V_1

    D. V_3, V_4

121. A patient in acute hepatic failure following toxic ingestion is admitted to the critical care unit. Expected lab changes include:

    A. Hyperkalemia and hypophosphatemia

    B. Hypokalemia and hypophosphatemia

    C. Hypokalemia and hypermagnesemia

    D. Hyperkalemia and hypomagnesemia

122. Which of the following are symptoms of spinal shock?

A. Constipation, low hematocrit, hyperglycemia

B. Urinary retention, hypotension, bradycardia

C. Weakness, tachycardia, hypertension

D. Irregular respiratory patterns in breathing, hyperglycemia, tachycardia

123. Which of the following murmurs is best heard with the bell of the stethoscope?

A. Mitral regurgitation

B. Split heart sounds

C. Aortic regurgitation

D. Aortic stenosis

124. The nurse is precepting a new graduate nurse in the care of a patient admitted to the PCU after right and left heart catheterization with arterial and venous sheaths in place. Which statement by the nurse demonstrates an understanding of care management in regards to sheath removal for this patient?

A. Discontinue the venous sheath first as time to hemostasis is shorter

B. Discontinue the arterial sheath first as the venous sheath may be vital in an emergency

C. Discontinue the arterial sheath to reduce the risk of DVT

D. Discontinue the venous sheath to minimize fistula formation

125. A patient is admitted for treatment of acute ischemia to the right leg requiring surgical embolectomy. During the procedure extra dye is used for arteriography. Post-op the patient is anuric. Which of the following immediate treatments should the nurse expect?

    A. Vasodilators

    B. Vasopressors

    C. Fluid challenge

    D. Dopamine

You can do it!

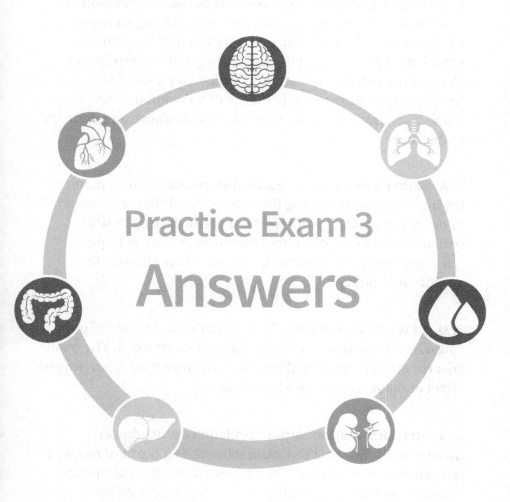

Practice Exam 3
Answers

Practice Exam #3 Answers with rationales

1. **B. Spiral CT/Angio scan to rule out pulmonary embolism.**
Shortness of breath, chest pain, and right calf/leg pain are all symptoms of a lower extremity DVT and acute pulmonary embolism. Spiral CT/Angio is the best option to visualize the clot and plan interventions accordingly. An elevated D-dimer level can help confirm the presence of a thrombus somewhere in the body, but is not specific enough to diagnose a pulmonary embolism.

2. **A. Gather more data about the infections.** Clinical inquiry begins with understanding the issue at hand. The staff need to figure out what type of infections are occurring in which patients before they can either formulate a clinical inquiry question, engage in education, or make other changes to practice and policy.

3. **D. ↑ Liver function tests.** Both enalapril and labetalol can cause hepatic injury, so elevated LFTs are a concern. The main adverse effect of both medications is hypotension; other adverse effect of enalapril includes hyperkalemia.

4. **A. Atrial fibrillation.** Atrial fibrillation occurs due to distension of the atrial myocardial tissue as a result of reduced left ventricular emptying. The tissues around the pulmonary veins are typical sites for atrial ectopy. 2nd degree AV block type II and 3rd degree AV block are complications associated with occlusion of the left anterior descending artery during acute coronary syndrome. 2nd degree AV block type I is seen with conditions that produce ischemia to the AV node.

5. **B. Anion gap: 10; urine ketone: negative; serum potassium: 5.3; blood glucose 850 mg/dL.** HHS does not produce an abnormal anion gap nor ketones. Patients presenting with hyperglycemic, hyperosmolar non-ketotic syndrome (HHS) are Type II diabetics. In Type II diabetes, the presence of endogenous insulin prevents a patient from developing ketosis and acidosis.

6. **A. Antero-septal-lateral.** There is ST elevation in leads V_1–V_6 and I & aVL. V_1–V_4 assess the anterior-septal wall which is perfused by the left anterior descending artery. Leads V_5, V_6, I & aVL assess the low and high lateral wall of the left ventricle which is normally perfused by the left circumflex artery. Because all walls appear to be affected, a high proximal occlusion in the left main artery should be suspected.

7. **A. Epinephrine 0.3 mg IM.** Angioedema, as evidenced by tongue swelling and breathing difficulty, is a sign of anaphylaxis and calls for immediate treatment with epinephrine. The patient could be having a reaction to the dye or another medication received during the process. The concentration of epinephrine used in anaphylaxis is 1:1000 vs. code dose epinephrine, which is 1:10,000. In addition to the administration of epinephrine, histamine blockers should be considered. H1 blockers such as diphenhydramine and H2 blockers such as ranitidine should be considered to block the release of histamine.

8. **A. At the left mid-clavicular line, during diastole.** The best place to auscultate the mitral valve is the left mid-clavicular line, 5th ICS-directly over the anatomic location of the valve. The mitral valve is open during diastole, so altered flow due to stenosis is best heard then.

9. **C. Prolonged QT interval.** Haloperidol is known to lengthen the QT interval and can lead to polymorphic ventricular tachycardia in susceptible patients. QTc monitoring is imperative, particularly for a patient receiving frequent or escalating doses of Haldol.

10. **B. Metabolic alkalosis.** When there is severe loss of gastric content as in the case of vomiting, there is also loss of hydrochloric acid (HCl). Whenever a hydrogen ion is lost, a bicarbonate ion is gained. In the setting of hypokalemia, alkalosis may be present due to intracellular shifting of bicarb ions. Other causes of metabolic alkalosis include diarrhea, excessive bicarbonate administration and excessive loop diuretic use.

11. **C. "I see the name Paul is listed on your name band, what name do you prefer to be called?"** In response to diversity it is vital to avoid assumptions in the care of a transgendered patient and ask them how they prefer to be addressed and the name they prefer to use.

12. **B. Inferior wall.** Leads II, III, and aVF trace electrical activity coming from the direction of the arms and center of the chest down toward the feet, and therefore give the most accurate picture of the inferior wall of the heart. Reciprocal changes are often seen in leads I & aVL.

13. **D. Hypomagnesemia.** Hypomagnesemia is a precipitant of Torsades de Pointes as it prolongs the QT interval. This is often seen in patients with chronic alcohol abuse. You may also see Torsades de Pointes referred to as polymorphic ventricular tachycardia. Numerous medications may induce Torsades de Pointes. These include antidepressants, phenothiazines, some

anti-viral and anti-fungal medications as well as all class Ia, Ic or III antiarrhythmic medications.

14. C. Hypovolemic shock. Patients with Diabetes Insipidus (DI) have profound fluid loss because of a lack of antidiuretic hormone (ADH). A S_3 heart sound would be auscultated in heart failure. Diabetes Insipidus does not cause dysrhythmias or adrenal crisis.

15. A. Severe sepsis. This patient is exhibiting signs of SIRS (T > 38° C and HR > 90) AND is likely to have infection due to the wounds and fractures. Additionally, the patient is now showing signs of hypoperfusion with decreased urine output. The confusion is a sign of organ dysfunction. Together, these clinical indicators put the patient in the category of severe sepsis; 2 or more SIRS + suspicion of infection + organ dysfunction.

16. C. Atrial fibrillation. In mitral insufficiency, blood flows backward into the left atrium. Depending on the blood volume, distention of the left atrium occurs over time, stretching inter-nodal pathways from the right atrium to left atrium, causing them to become dysfunctional. Over time this can lead to atrial fibrillation.

17. C. Calcium channel blockers & beta blockers. In hypertrophic cardiomyopathy, the ventricular septum is thickened and enlarged. Beta blockers help slow or reverse the ventricular dysfunction; and calcium channel blockers help ease outflow tract obstruction and symptoms such as arrhythmias and dyspnea. Both medications slow the heart rate allowing for maximal filling in a reduced left ventricle. Both may also help prevent sudden cardiac death.

18. **D. Diabetic ulcer.** Diabetic ulcers usually appear on the plantar aspect of the foot, over metatarsal heads, or under the heel with diminished or absent sensation in the foot with well-defined wound margins, possible cellulitis. Variable amounts of exudate, possible necrosis and tissue granulation.

19. **D. Collaborate with the provider to minimize delirium inducing medications and develop a plan to facilitate sleep.** Delirium increases the risk of mortality and morbidity, minimizing the use of delirium inducing medications and developing a plan of care to facilitate sleep is most appropriate. Restraints can increase the severity of experiences by a delirious patient.

20. **A. A mental health disorder that is triggered by a terrifying event.** Post-traumatic stress disorder (PTSD) is a mental health condition that is triggered by a terrifying event, either experiencing it or witnessing the event. PTSD may occur following critical life-threatening illness. The signs and symptoms may include; severe anxiety, nightmares/night terrors, flashbacks, tachycardia, restlessness, and hyperventilation. PTSD usually responds to psychotherapy and medications.

21. **C. Partially compensated respiratory acidosis.** The pH is low, indicating acidosis, and the $PaCO_2$ is elevated, indicating hypercapnia and hypoventilation indicating a respiratory source. Because the bicarb is also elevated, we know that compensation has begun, so this is a partially compensated respiratory acidosis.

22. **B. Frequent electrolyte monitoring to identify electrolyte shifts.** Intermittent hemodialysis removes large amounts of fluid, electrolytes and waste over a short period of time. Electrolytes can shift rapidly, including calcium, potassium,

and sodium. Impacts can be significant if not followed closely for the cardiovascular, respiratory, and neurologic systems. Hemodynamic monitoring can be helpful though not necessarily a priority in a hemodynamically stable patient. Decisions for continuing or stopping HD are not based on urine output production alone. Weight monitoring is important though on a daily basis and frequent electrolyte monitoring is a greater priority.

23. **A. Ask the patient if he likes music & what type.** Before beginning music therapy or any complementary or alternative therapy, it's essential to know if the patient likes what the therapy involves! Playing music that is not what the patient enjoys may increase stress and depression.

24. **C. Synchronized cardioversion with 100 joules.** New onset, rapid atrial fibrillation that is symptomatic with unstable vital signs calls for immediate synchronized cardioversion. Pharmacologic rate control should be initiated if attempts to cardiovert are unsuccessful. Chronic atrial fibrillation should not be cardioverted unless a transthoracic echocardiogram or transesophageal echocardiogram have been performed to rule out cardiac thrombus. Rapid atrial fibrillation that is chronic should be rate controlled with medications versus cardioverted.

25. **A. Standing behind organizational decisions that are formed based on the needs of patients.** Standing behind organizational decisions that foster the needs of your patient is an example of advocacy. Working with individuals to create synergistic relationships is an example of collaboration. Consistently acting with intention and upholding ethical values and principles is an example of accountability. Being an honest and trustworthy individual is an example of integrity.

26. **A. Tracheal deviation to the left and absent breath sounds over the pneumothorax.** A right-sided pneumothorax will exert pressure on the right lung and eventually force it and the upper airways and trachea to the opposite direction. Since no air is moving in and out of lungs with a pneumothorax, breath sounds are absent.

27. **D. Subdural hematoma.** A subdural bleed is usually a slow accumulating, venous bleed. Abnormal neuro changes may not be seen for days or weeks. Epidural hematomas may bleed and accumulate rapidly since they result from arterial bleeding. Cerebral aneurysm rupture is associated with the patient complaining of the "worst headache of her life" (thunderclap headache). Arteriovenous malformations are congenital and do not result from a fall.

28. **C. Delirium.** The Confusion Assessment Method scale (CAM) is a useful tool in identifying cognitive impairment or delirium. The CAM assesses four features: acute change or fluctuation in mental status from baseline, inattention, altered level of consciousness and disorganized thinking. The CAM is not used to assess Post-traumatic Stress Disorder, dementia or depression.

29. **B. Sulfa-trimethoprim (Bactrim).** Anemia can be caused or exacerbated by some medications, including sulfa-trimethoprim, other antibiotics, and ACE-inhibitors. Beta-blocking agents and diuretics don't contribute to anemia, and EPO may be used to treat anemia. This patient may have long standing anemia, but antibiotic treatment may be tailored to avoid exacerbation.

30. **C. 2nd degree AV block type II.** 1st and 3rd degree AV block have regular ventricular rhythms. In the 2nd degree Type II, the ventricular rhythm is irregular due to a dropped QRS-complex.

In 2nd degree AV block type I, the PR-interval progressively lengthens whereas in 2nd degree AV block type II, the PR-interval remains constant when a QRS complex is present.

31. **D. V$_3$ & V$_4$.** Leads I, aVL, V$_5$ & V$_6$ view the high and low lateral wall. Leads II, III & aVF view the inferior wall. V$_1$ & V$_2$ assess the interventricular septum. Many times leads V$_1$ through V$_4$ are referred to as the antero-septal leads.

32. **C. Calcium.** Diphenhydramine is a histamine-1 receptor blocker. Glucagon is the appropriate antidote for beta-blocker toxicity. Although it may be tempting to choose atropine because of the bradycardia, atropine is not the antidote and will not likely increase the heart rate until the antidote is administered.

33. **A. Lipase & amylase and a bolus of IV fluids.** Patients that are severely dehydrated are at risk of developing acute pancreatitis. Pancreatitis is an inflammation of the pancreas that affects insulin levels. Stabbing pain, dehydration, and mottled skin are common signs. Lipase, amylase, and serum glucose should be ordered. All three would be elevated in pancreatitis. The patient should be NPO during the acute phase of pancreatitis as food will exacerbate the pancreatic pain. With that said, it is important to provide nutrition as early as possible. If needed, a small bore, distal feeding tube can be placed past the pancreatic duct.

34. **B. Pulmonary embolism.** With an anterior wall MI, tachycardia and a wet sounding cough may be part of the clinical assessment profile. However, given with the history of a complicated abdominal surgery and two days of immobilization, suspicion for pulmonary embolism should be high. Clinical signs including anxiety and sudden onset shortness of breath points to a priority to rule out pulmonary embolism.

35. **B. Use a certified translation service.** Use of a certified translation service is the most appropriate way to communicate with patients who do not speak English. They are trained and certified to translate medical information without bias. The patient's family may not know how to translate some medical terms and may not translate certain information to the patient or nurse in the best interest of the patient. Translation mobile applications are not completely accurate and may not be able to translate medical terms appropriately. Closed-ended questions are never appropriate when communicating with patients as it limits the patient with providing the healthcare team important information.

36. **C. Decreased albumin, elevated amylase & lipase.** Elevated amylase is a hallmark sign of acute pancreatitis, although the level doesn't predict the severity of the disease. Lipase is also elevated and will remain elevated for a longer period of time. In pancreatitis, inflammation leads to vasodilation and extravasation of albumin; poor nutritional status also contributes to hypoalbuminemia.

37. **C. Furosemide 20 mg IV x 1.** The patient is admitted with decompensated heart failure. A S3 heart sound and crackles are indicative of fluid overload. Therefore, a diuretic would be appropriate at this time.

38. **A. Call for help and prepare to transcutaneous pace.** Transcutaneous pacing is the treatment of choice for 2nd degree AV block type II as well as 3rd degree AV block. Atropine administration may not be effective due to the block occurring lower in the conduction system at the His-Purkinje fiber level. Defibrillation is not appropriate. Calling the provider is appropriate; however, the unstable nature of the patient requires immediate intervention with a transcutaneous pacemaker.

39. D. Vitamin K. Warfarin (Coumadin) is a vitamin K antagonist, so the best way to reverse it is administration of vitamin K. If other coagulopathies exist, those could be treated with platelets, protamine, or cryoprecipitate as indicated. Fresh frozen plasma (FFP) may also be considered.

40. C. Ask the patient what they already know about diabetes. It's best to assess what the patient already knows about the disease. This allows you to focus on correcting any information they provided that was inaccurate and focus on knowledge gaps about the disease, rather than focusing on information they already know that is accurate.

Patients with a new diagnosis may not be able to process all the information you had provided them. It is important to provide education in small doses. Written information is a good modality for patient to learn; however, many patients need a variety of learning modalities to retain the information. Eventually it is important for the patient to inject themselves by returning demonstration with direct focused feedback; however, this is not the best when first assessing the best way to educate the patient.

41. D. "Palliative care is a great resource to support your goals for treatment and quality of life as you make decisions about your care." Nursing opportunity for education includes active listening about fears, provision of empathy, and education about how coordination of care can be facilitated with Palliative care.

42. A. Keep the patient's head in a neutral midline position. A neutral midline position promotes venous drainage thereby preventing or decreasing intracranial pressure (ICP). You should only keep the HOB flat for hemodynamic instability. Otherwise the HOB should be elevated to promote venous drainage. Hyperthermia increases metabolic demands, which may in turn raise ICP.

43. B. Beta$_2$ agonist. Immediate treatment of asthma exacerbation is to bronchodilate the airways to facilitate ventilation. Beta$_2$ agonists such as albuterol are a mainstay in the management of asthma and can be administered via continuous nebulizer if needed.

44. B. Acute Respiratory Distress Syndrome. Criteria for ARDS include bilateral pulmonary infiltrates on chest x-ray and a P/F ratio ≤ 300; it is further rated as mild-moderate-severe based on P/F ratio. To calculate the P/F ratio, divide the PaO$_2$ by the FiO$_2$. In this case $102 \div 1.0 = 102$, making it borderline severe ARDS. Pneumonia placed the patient at risk for developing ARDS.

45. B. Loop diuretics. Hypokalemia is common with loop diuretics and a state of alkalosis. Patients that are dehydrated are acidotic which causes hyperkalemia as the hydrogen ions decrease causing cellular polarity to maintain by retaining potassium. Patients may develop hyperkalemia when receiving a blood transfusion.

46. B. Haloperidol. Haloperidol is the agent of choice for delirium treatment, although the evidence is limited. Newer studies are questioning whether any medication is effective in the treatment of delirium. There is newer, limited evidence that Precedex (dexmetotomidine) may be more helpful than antipsychotic medications such as Haldol. Benzodiazepines worsen delirium and should be avoided.

47. C. NIHSS. The National Institute of Health Stroke Scale (NIHSS) evaluates severity of debilitation after stroke and predicts recoverability. Hunt and Hess is used to grade subarachnoid hemorrhage, CPSS (Cincinnati Pre-hospital Stroke Scale) is used to identify stroke. MEND (Miami Emergency Neurologic Deficit) takes features from CPSS and NIHSS and is used as a communication tool. MEND is similar to GCS but more specific for stroke.

48. **C. Thromboxane A$_2$.** Acetylsalicylic acid inhibits the release of Thromboxane A$_2$ from the endothelium. Thromboxane A$_2$ reacts with platelets to activate them and initiate clot formation. Patients on acetylsalicylic acid (aspirin) may be at higher risk for bleeding since platelet activation is altered resulting in decreased platelet aggregation, preventing clot formation. The effects of Nitric Oxide are vasodilatation and neurotransmission. Medications such as nitroglycerin and amyl nitrite serve as vasodilators because they are converted to nitric oxide in the body.

49. **C. Increased risk of infection, bleeding and anemia.** The clinical manifestations of transplant failure are similar to the initial signs and symptoms of leukemia; increased risk of infection because of lowered white cell count, bleeding as a result of pancytopenia and anemia due to low hemoglobin count from bleeding.

50. **B. Relieve portal venous pressure.** Trans-jugular intrahepatic portal shunt (TIPS) is an interventional radiology procedure where a shunt is placed to bypass the liver. The shunt goes from the portal vein, which feeds blood into the liver, to one of the hepatic veins, which carry blood back to the vena cava. Pressure in the portal vein decreases and with it the congestion and backup such as esophageal varices are also improved.

51. **C. 2nd degree Type II.** In 2nd degree type II heart block, conduction of the cardiac impulse is blocked below the AV node in the bundle or branches. The Bundle of His lies directly in the anterior wall so is most likely to be affected.

52. **C. Emboli.** Endocarditis with an infectious source will often lead to bacteria building up on the endocardium. On echocardiogram, the bacteria looks like a long strand of yarn being moved by blood flow through the heart. One of the risks of infective endocarditis is the strand breaking and throwing bacterial emboli forward into the lungs (from the right heart) or the brain/body (from the left heart).

53. **A. Review prescribed medications with the provider in daily rounds.** Patients with GERD are generally prescribed a stomach acid blocker. A lower gastric pH can decrease the effectiveness of the ampicillin. The most appropriate next step for the RN is to review the medication list and interactions with the providers and pharmacists to ensure patient safety.

54. **B. Fluid removal only.** In the setting of ATN, the goal of therapy is to remove excess fluid, maintain optimal electrolyte balance, remove waste and correct acid/base imbalance, namely acidosis. The term ultrafiltration refers to removal of fluid. Ultrafiltration promotes fluid removal by using hydrostatic pressure to force fluid against a semi-permeable membrane. Removal of cytokines from septic patient or to decrease the serum osmolality is not the primary indication for use for hemodialysis, however, is ideal to remove excess fluid to stabilize the patient's fluid balance.

55. **C. Left-sided pronator drift.** Headache, drowsiness, and mild memory loss or confusion can be side effects of anesthesia that persist for several hours. Pronator drift indicates focal motor weakness and may be a sign of compromised neurological function following surgery.

56. **A. Drain serosanguinous drainage post-op.** Unlike a chest tube used for pneumothorax or hemothorax, where the focus

is improved lung expansion, chest tubes in cardiac surgery patients are used as postop drains. They are located in the mediastinal space rather than the pleural space and therefore have no pulmonary function.

57. **C. Prevention of the spread of the virus.** Although the other items are important and included in the care of the patient with Hepatitis C, prevention of the spread of the virus is vital for the safety of the caregiver and other patients in the unit.

58. **C. A calcium channel-blocking agent.** Calcium channel blockers act on the coronary arteries, causing vasodilation and relief of coronary vasospasm. Beta-blockers have a less specific effect on the peripheral vascular system. Cholinergic agents vasodilate but have other unwanted effects on the cardiopulmonary system.

59. **A. Call for help and immediately start CPR.** The rhythm is ventricular fibrillation and requires immediate CPR and defibrillation. First, call for help and the defibrillator. Then, perform CPR until the defibrillator is present, prepared, charged, and ready to deliver the countershock. Synchronized cardioversion is not an appropriate treatment modality for ventricular fibrillation. Medication administration is not proper at this time in the advanced life support treatment algorithm.

60. **B. Hypoactive bowel sounds & leukocytosis.** Infarcted bowel slows or stops motility throughout the gut, and causes an immune inflammatory response that leads to leukocytosis.

61. **D. STAT serum lactate and blood cultures.** The patient is experiencing sepsis. The patient has a suspected infection and there are at least 4 SIRS criteria that have been met. According to the Surviving Sepsis campaign, the presence of organ

dysfunction is determined by acquisition of a STAT serum lactate. Additionally, blood cultures can be drawn at this time as part of the sepsis bundle. Antibiotic administration and fluid resuscitation should be prioritized if infection is suspected.

62. **C. Potential for infection.** Bilateral periorbital ecchymosis (Raccoon's eyes) and bruising at the mastoid bone (Battle sign) in association with head injury indicate a disruption in the dura mater. Blood and/or CSF may leak from the ear or nose (Otorrhea or rhinorrhea). These openings may serve as a portal of entry for bacteria and the potential for a CNS infection.

63. **B. RR 20 with shallow breathing and decreased LOC.** In a patient with respiratory distress, a sudden decrease in respiratory rate indicates exhaustion and impending respiratory failure. Changes in work of breathing and saturation may also be present, but don't necessarily indicate an emergent need for intubation.

64. **A. Shortened QT interval on ECG.** Signs and symptoms of hypercalcemia occur when the calcium level is greater than 11 mg/dL. Hypercalcemia can cause abnormal heart rhythms and shortened QT intervals and ST segments. A positive Chvostek or Trousseau sign would be present with hypocalcemia. Grey-Turner's sign refers to flank bruising, which correlates with pancreatitis or retroperitoneal bleeding, not hypercalcemia.

65. **A. Provide a private quiet room so they can spend time alone.** Families need time to absorb bad news, deal with their initial emotions, and grieve together. Once they have had time together, they can be involved and assisted with specific tasks.

66. **D. Normal saline boluses.** During and after right ventricular (RV) infarction, the right side of the heart is dependent on adequate filling pressures (preload) to maintain adequate

cardiac output. Small boluses of normal saline should be administered and titrated to achieve optimal output before any other medications are considered. Preload reducing medications such as nitroglycerin, morphine, beta blockers and diuretics should be avoided as they may lower the blood pressure. Often in right ventricular MI, the wall motion is stunned, negatively affecting forward flow of blood to the left ventricle.

67. **A. Ondansetron.** A prolonged QT interval in males is defined as ≥ 450 ms, so certain medications should be administered with caution or held until the provider is notified. Common medications that prolong QT interval include: Antiarrhythmic agents: Class IA, IB, III, tricyclic antidepressants, phenothiazine, macrolide antimicrobials (especially Erythromycin), Nicardipine, Cisapride and haloperidol.

68. **C. Watch for signs of hypoglycemia.** Because food intake is drastically decreased immediately after gastric bypass, patients with type II diabetes may have decreased blood sugars. As weight is lost and insulin resistance decreases, the blood sugars may normalize and allow a medication-dependent patient to rely on diet alone to control levels.

69. **C. File a safety report and bring it to the attention of nursing leadership.** The most appropriate step by the nurse is to report the objective findings and bring it to the attention of leadership to review the cases, determine the root cause, determine if there are other cases in the organization, and bring in resources for next steps. Blame of the previous nurse is not helpful and stopping using the product is not the appropriate next step.

70. **B. Muffled heart sounds, tachycardia with hypotension and jugular vein distention.** The clinical manifestations of a cardiac

tamponade is denoted by Beck's Triad, which consists of muffled heart sounds, tachycardia with hypotension and jugular vein distention. In addition, the central venous pressure (right heart preload) will be elevated and the pulse pressure (systole minus diastole) will be narrow. Normal pulse pressure is 40 mm Hg.

Muffled heart sounds are caused by the fluid accumulation in the pericardial sac, the narrowing pulse pressure and hypotension are caused from the increasing pressure outside of the heart during diastole. The JVD is caused by the backup of blood into the venous system on the right side of the heart.

71. **A. If they have a specific plan to attempt suicide again.** You will need to assess if the patient has intent or a plan to cause harm to themselves. If so, they will need to be on active suicide precautions.

72. **D. Cool, pale, moist skin.** Cardiogenic shock results from the impaired ability of the ventricle to pump blood forward, which leads to a decrease in Stroke Volume (SV) and an increase in left end diastolic volume (LEDV). The decrease in SV activates the RASS system resulting in vasoconstriction, which causes in an increased systemic vasculature resistance. The increase in LEDV results in an increased left ventricular preload, which manifests as pulmonary congestion and crackles. This pulmonary edema causes impaired gas exchange and impaired tissue perfusion resulting in cool, pale, moist skin. You would not expect to hear wheezes with pulmonary edema. This would be more common in a restrictive airway disease.

73. **A. Purpura and petechiae.** Disseminated intravascular coagulation (DIC) is a systemic activation of blood coagulation resulting in a deposition of fibrin causing a microvascular thrombi in organs. This often leads to multiple organ dysfunction syndrome (MODS) due to hypoperfusion.

Consumption and subsequent exhaustion of coagulation proteins and platelets may induce severe bleeding. Oozing and bleeding is an indication of DIC, often with a platelet count less than 100,000.

74. D. The patient's ability to be alert and follow commands. The safety of early mobilization in patients with multiple tubes and lines, including endotracheal tubes, has been established in the critical care nursing literature. The most important factor in determining the level of mobility (e.g. up to chair vs ambulation) is the patient's level of consciousness and ability to follow commands.

75. D. Elevated pulmonary artery pressure. Pulmonary arterial hypertension can manifest with clinical indications of right ventricular failure and hemodynamic parameters including pulmonary vascular resistance (PVR) > 250, resting mean pulmonary arterial pressure > 25 mm Hg and a normal left atrial pressure (preload) < 15 mm Hg. In addition, the right atrial pressure or preload will be elevated as well. While performing a right heart catheterization, often an acute pulmonary vasodilator challenge is administered to determine the presence of vaso-reactivity. Treatment of idiopathic pulmonary arterial hypertension includes pulmonary vasodilators such as sildenafil or Bosentan. More aggressive treatment includes a continuous infusion of Epoprostenol (Flolan) or Remodulin.

76. B. D-dimer 650 ng/mL. D-dimer is formed and elevates when plasmin degrades cross-linked fibrin, as in the presence of an embolism, so the level will be elevated with venous thromboembolism (VTE). In low to moderate risk patients, a negative D-dimer can actually rule out VTE. Other levels may be abnormal depending on the comorbidities or treatments being used.

77. D. Mallory-Weiss Tear. A Mallory-Weiss Tear is a complication from severe vomiting in different populations of individuals. Most tears heal on their own, though endoscopic evaluation may be required.

78. C. U waves. Hypokalemia secondary to diuresis can lead to impaired myocardial conduction and prolonged ventricular repolarization. This is evident by bradycardia, flattened T waves, and prominent u waves. Peaked T waves and a widened QRS would be secondary to hyperkalemia.

79. D. S_3. The S_3 heart sound is heard when there is decreased ventricular compliance. As blood is ejected from the atria, the rate of flow slows as it hits the distended or stiff ventricle and causes S_3. A S_4 heart sound would be auscultated in patients with increased resistance like left ventricular hypertrophy or in an acute myocardial infarction. A split S_1 would be heard with a bundle branch block or PVCs. A pericardial friction rub would be auscultated in the setting of pericarditis.

80. C. IV fluids. In the contused heart, preload needs to be optimized to ensure adequate cardiac output. Since the inflammatory response to trauma also involves vasodilation and relative or actual hypovolemia, IV fluids are the most appropriate choice. If the patient continues with hypotension and signs of hypoperfusion, an echocardiogram should be performed to assess left ventricular function and rule out cardiac tamponade.

81. A. Administer diphenhydramine (Benadryl) 25 mg IV push. Haldol can cause dystonic reactions such as tremors, slurred speech, and torticollis, all of which should be treated with Benadryl. Anti-seizure medications are not appropriate, and a more complete stroke assessment should preclude calling the stroke team. Flumazenil is the antidote for lorazepam (Ativan) and is not useful in this situation.

82. **D. Turn the patient to their side and set up suction equipment.** The first action for a patient experiencing seizure is to assess and manage airway. Oral airways may injure the patient or stimulate a gag reflex, so positioning and ensuring suction is available are the first actions. An anti-seizure medication may be indicated, but should be administered intravenously or intramuscularly until the patient is awake and able to take oral medications safely.

83. **C. Hepato-Jugular reflex sign.** Bibasilar crackles are noted in patients with left-sided heart failure from fluid in the lungs causing an increase in opacities in a Chest x-ray Pitting edema and hepato-jugular vein distention are noted in right-sided heart failure. To assess for hepato-jugular vein distention, sit the patient up at a 30–45 degree angle, have them turn their head to the left and perform deep palpation in the RUQ of the abdomen around the border of the liver. Compression is usually done for less than 20 seconds. If the jugular veins distend, that is a sign of right sided heart congestion. You may notice that the liver is enlarged during deep palpation.

84. **D. Warfarin, furosemide, and amlodipine**. Long-term anticoagulation, diuretics, and calcium channel blockers in responsive patients are part of the standard medication regimen in pulmonary hypertension. Beta-blockers are contraindicated as they may decrease right-sided heart function.

85. **B. Assessing comfort.** Obtaining consent and determining code status are legal activities that require a professional translator. Discharge planning is also complex and may require an interpreter who understands medical jargon. While a formal nursing assessment should include a translator, the family is often able to help determine if the patient is comfortable.

86. **D. Tachycardia, Hypotension, Hyperthermia.** During the compensatory stage of septic shock, there is an inflammatory response leading to peripheral arterial vasodilation and capillary leak. This leads to hypoperfusion from hypotension induced intravascular volume depletion. As a compensatory reaction when stroke volume drops, the heart rate increases as evidenced by tachycardia to improve O_2 supply due to increased demands. Septic patients are often febrile and hyperthermic but can become hypothermic in the late stages of septic shock. Early recognition and initiation of fluid resuscitation and antimicrobial administration in the first hours is crucial.

87. **C. Furosemide (Lasix) 40 mg IV and a Dobutamine infusion at 2.5 mcg/kg/min.** Cardiogenic shock is caused by an inability of the heart to pump effectively. Clinical manifestations of cardiogenic shock include poor tissue perfusion, anxiety, and fluid overload with elevated preload, low cardiac output and increased afterload. Collaborative management includes reducing preload (diuresis) and increasing contractility (Dobutamine). Blood pressure may be supported with a vasopressor such as norepinephrine (Levophed). If this therapy does not improve the hemodynamics, the patient should be transferred to the ICU where mechanical support such as an intra-aortic balloon pump or Impella ventricular assist device should be considered.

88. **D. Inspection, auscultation, palpation.** The abdominal exam should proceed from least invasive to most invasive so that percussion or palpations do not trigger bowel sounds that weren't already there. Palpating the abdomen is always the last step in the abdominal examination. An easy way to remember this is "look, listen, feel"; Inspection, auscultation, percussion & palpation.

89. **D. Bradycardia, systolic hypertension, wide pulse pressure.** As intracranial pressure increases, cerebral vessels

vasoconstrict to maintain cerebral blood flow. Compression upon the pons and upper medulla affect the cardiac and vasomotor centers. Bradycardia and systolic hypertension occur.

90. B. Administer Glucagon 3 mg IV. Glucagon is used in beta-blocker overdose because it increases heart rate and works outside of the beta-adrenergic receptor function. Atropine will increase the rate of p waves, but does not help conduction in 2nd degree type 2 heart block.

91. D. Motor response, verbal response, eye opening. The function of the GCS is to provide information about head injured or comatose patients over time, allowing for recognition of changes for the worse and improvements. It also allows researchers to compare outcomes amongst head injury patients with similar injuries or scores at the time of admission.

92. A. Calcium. Calcium citrate is used as a preservative in banked blood, but binds with calcium in the body. Hypocalcemia is a common complication of transfusion, especially with large volumes of PRBCs, so ionized calcium levels should be closely monitored.

93. B. Closure of the anion gap, maintaining serum K⁺ above 3.3 mEq/L, and decreasing of the blood glucose below 250 mg/dl. In the management of DKA as the acidosis is corrected the anion gap closes and the goal is prevent hypokalemia and lowering blood sugars slowly below 250 through fluid resuscitation, administration of KCL, and utilization of an insulin infusion.

94. B. Sodium replacement should not exceed 0.5 mEq/L per hour. Correcting the sodium level greater than 0.5 mEq/L/hour (12 mEq/L per day) have been associated with acute osmotic myelinolysis (demyelination syndrome). Infusion rates less than 50 ml/hr can be given via peripheral IV although central venous delivery is preferred. Therapy should continue within the above defined parameters until the serum sodium reaches 130 mEq/L. At that time, therapy should be discontinued to prevent hypernatremia.

95. **A. Helicobacter pylori.** Helicobacter pylori is a gram-negative bacteria found in the stomach. Overgrowth of this bacteria damages the gastric mucosa, leading to gastric ulcers.

96. **C. Place in reverse Trendelenburg & administer furosemide.** Positioning the patient so that the fluid (ascites) is not compressing his diaphragm will help his dyspnea. Diuresis is also necessary to help control the ascites.

97. **C. Increases oxygen requirements of the brain tissue.** An increase in temperature may increase intracranial pressure. Acetaminophen may not be effective if the elevated temperature is secondary to the brain injury. An elevation in systemic and brain temperature will result in an increase in oxygen demand of the brain tissue, when oxygen delivery is at risk. Fevers are often associated with worse neurologic outcomes in neurologically impaired patients.

98. **C. Low fiber, low dairy.** Patients recovering from a partial obstruction benefit from a low residual diet. A low fiber, low dairy diet allows the intestines to digest and absorb the food and nutrients more easily and leave little residual material for the digestive tract to process. High fiber and high protein foods may induce ketosis if combined with low carbohydrate intake.

99. **D. Hyperkalemia & hyponatremia.** Sodium is often low or normal upon presentation with DKA. Glucose has a

dilutional effect on the sodium. Potassium is often elevated due to intracellular shifting and from metabolic acidosis. Hyperkalemia and hyponatremia are early findings that correct once fluids and insulin are administered. Patients in DKA have an increase in plasma osmolality and low to normal phosphate levels initially. Ketones are present in the blood and urine, but will continue to spill in the urine beyond the point ketosis has been shut down in the serum.

100. **B. Position with the head of bed 30 degrees to optimize venous outflow.** Patient positioning is a first-line therapy for optimizing cerebral perfusion. Obstruction to venous outflow can immediately increase ICPs. Other therapies can be instituted as needed.

101. **D. Uncompensated metabolic acidosis with mild hypoxia.** The pH depicts a state of acidosis. The component that has moved in the same acid direction as the pH is the HCO_3. The $PaCO_2$ has not deviated from its normal range to compensate for the disturbance. Mild hypoxia is a PaO_2 from 60–80 mm Hg.

102. **C. Discuss assignments with the nurses involved.** A collaborative approach involving the affected nurses is the best way to build teamwork and promote a healthy work environment.

103. **B. Phenobarbital.** Phenobarbital is a barbiturate. If ingested in excessive amounts, causes bradycardia, hypotension, and stupor. Aspirin overdose leads to hyperventilation, hyperthermia, and coma. Excess alcohol intake can produce hypoventilation, tachycardia, and irritability. Cocaine ingestion causes tachycardia, hypertension, and tremors.

104. **D. Beta blockers.** Cocaine ingestion stimulates alpha and beta receptors. Physical signs and symptoms of cocaine toxicity include tachycardia, vasoconstriction induced hypertension, myocardial ischemia and hyperthermia. If beta blockers are administered in the setting of ischemia and infarction, this leaves unopposed alpha stimulation which can cause severe vasoconstriction and lead to hypertensive crisis and bleeding. In general, nitrates and calcium channel blockers are administered to vasodilate coronary arteries in the setting of a cocaine induced MI.

105. **A. Acute pericarditis.** Given the clinical picture—recent history of a myocardial infarction, presence of a pericardial friction run, non-responsiveness to nitroglycerin, positional pain and relief with NSAIDs, this all leads to suspicion of pericarditis. There is diffuse ST elevations in the inferior, anterior, septal and lateral leads. In the setting of inferior ST elevation (II, III, aVF), you would normally expect to observe ST depression or a reciprocal change in leads I & aVL. However, the ST segment is elevated in those leads.

106. **B. Hemodialysis.** For severe salicylate poisoning as well as methanol, ethylene glycol, and lithium overdose, hemodialysis is indicated. Gastric lavage or activated charcoal may provide some benefit if performed close to the time of ingestion. Sodium bicarb is useful in tricyclic antidepressant overdoses and maybe used in salicylate overdoses to alkinalize the urine. N-acetylcysteine is used for acetaminophen overdose.

107. **B. Forming clots when calcium reacts with Factor Xa.** Calcium is a byproduct of the parathyroid gland and is necessary for bone conservation and contraction of vascular smooth muscle. A sufficient level of combined Factor Xa and calcium is needed to form the final common pathway to produce clot formation. Many blood products have an added preservative

called citrate. Citrate binds with calcium, decreasing the available serum calcium.

108. **C. Excessive ADH.** Excessive ADH causes the kidneys to hold on to water thereby diluting the serum sodium level. A & B are both thyroid hormones having no impact on sodium levels.

109. **D. Right coronary artery.** The 12 Lead ECG reveals ST segment elevation in leads II, III and aVF. These leads assess the inferior wall of the left ventricle perfused by the right coronary artery. In addition, there is ST segment elevation in leads V_1–V_3. This is consistent with a right ventricular infarction. A right sided ECG should be performed to assess for elevation is V_R2–V_R4. The left anterior descending perfuses the anterior-septal wall, the left proximal perfuses the left lateral wall.

110. **B. Hypocalcemia & hyperglycemia.** Hypocalcemia and hyperglycemia are common problems in acute pancreatitis and require careful monitoring and treatment to maintain normal. Prolonged hyperglycemia can perpetuate a fluid deficit by causing an osmotic diuresis and hypocalcemia can impact cardiac function.

111. **B. 2nd ICS; left sternal border.** 2nd ICS, right sternal border is the aortic auscultation site. 3rd ICS, left sternal border is Erb's point. 5th ICS, midclavicular line is the mitral auscultation landmark.

112. **B. Pantoprazole 8 mg/hour IV infusion.** Prior to endoscopic evaluation proton pump inhibitors are used to decrease stomach acid and help stabilize a possible clot if an ulcer is suspected. IV fluids should also be started to maintain adequate intravascular volume.

113. B. Call for help, support airway/breathing, prepare to give Epinephrine (1:1000) 0.3 mg IM. The patient is having an anaphylactic reaction to contrast material. It is vital to summon additional assistance and support the airway since the patient could go into respiratory distress at any moment. Diphenhydramine would not be an appropriate intervention for anaphylaxis. It is given to block secondary effects of histamine. Intravenous doses of epinephrine are not the appropriate route of administration. One mg dosing of epinephrine is used for cardiac arrest intervention. Epinephrine (1:1000) 0.3 mg IM is the correct dose.

114. B. Partially compensated respiratory acidosis. This is a typical blood gas in a decompensated COPD patient. The patient is hypercapnic evidenced by the elevated $PaCO_2$. The elevated $PaCO_2$ causes the pH to drop, leading to a respiratory acidosis (low pH, elevated $PaCO_2$). The kidneys attempt to compensate by producing HCO_3, however it is not working in this case. The HCO_3 is leaning toward alkalosis. Because of this it is a partially compensated respiratory acidosis.

115. A. Alteplase (Activase) 100 mg IV over 2 hours. Sepsis is a prothrombotic state. The immediate and sudden change in respiratory compliance coupled with hypoxia should lead the nurse to suspect pulmonary embolism. Appropriate treatment for hemodynamically unstable PE is fibrinolytic treatment.

116. D. Hyperkalemia. In the setting of hyperkalemia (K+ > 5.5) a variety of ECG changes may be observed, depending on the potassium level. Common early ECG changes include T wave peaking. QRS widening, P wave widening and the loss of the PR interval are all associated with higher levels of potassium. In extreme hyperkalemia, patients may develop a sine wave, which exhibits as bradycardia with wide QRS complexes. ECG changes associated with hypomagnesemia and hypokalemia include prolongation of the QT interval, ST segment depression and the development of U waves.

117. A. Convene inter-professional team to review missing required patient education and establish standard processes for documentation of discharge education. Patient education needs to be inter-professional to be successful in both the evaluation of learning and ensuring that all points of discharge teaching are covered collaborations from all professionals will make it the most successful. Standardization of expected documentation ensures expectations are clear, increases accountability, and makes auditing and follow through to the standard possible.

118. C. Transfusion of platelets & cryoprecipitate. In DIC, the treatment priority is to replace clotting factors and mitigate bleeding while fixing the underlying problem. In this case the underlying problem is sepsis. Other conditions that put a patient at risk for DIC include obstetric emergencies and trauma.

119. A. 18-year-old traumatic brain injury. ADH is formed in the hypothalamus of the brain. Patients with head injuries or those undergoing organ donation are at risk for developing Diabetes Insipidus because of brain injury.

120. B. I, aVL. Leads II, III, and aVF reflect electrical activity in the inferior wall of the left ventricle. Leads I and aVL show reciprocal activity in the inferior from a different direction, so they will also show changes when the inferior wall is affected. I & aVL are sensitive reciprocal leads for inferior wall MIs.

121. A. Hypokalemia and hypophosphatemia. Along with elevated liver enzymes, typical electrolyte changes in hepatic failure include hypokalemia, hypophosphatemia, hypomagnesemia, and hypocalcemia.

122. **A. Urinary retention, hypotension, bradycardia.** Spinal shock refers to impaired functions of the spinal cord, usually due to inflammation. This can result in a temporary loss of reflexes just below the level of the injury. In acute spinal shock, there is a vasodilatory response. Bradycardia and cardiac dysthymias are often observed due to impairment of the autonomic nervous control system.

Motor paralysis, weakness, incoordination, and urine retention are commonly seen after an acute spinal injury, however, gradual recovery of these reflexes will occur once the compression or swelling has decreased. An elevated WBC would indicate an infection, which is not a common symptom of spinal shock.

123. **D. Aortic stenosis.** The bell of the stethoscope is best for listening to low frequency sounds. Examples of low frequency heart sounds include S1, S3, S4 and murmurs of stenosis. I always remember the be**LL** is used to listen to **L**ow pitched sounds.

124. **B. Discontinue the arterial sheath first as the venous sheath may be vital in an emergency.** Though the time to hemostasis is shorter with a venous sheath, if there is a complication in the removal of the arterial sheath the venous sheath can be used for blood administration or vasopressor administration.

125. **C. Fluid challenge.** Intrarenal failure occurs when there is damage to the functional units of the kidney by contrast dye, medications, or other toxins. Diuretics are used to help stimulate kidney function. In the setting of contrast induced nephropathy, IV fluids are key. Ideally fluids would be given prior to dye load. A saying I always remember: "The solution to pollution (contrast) is dilution!" The evidence to support sodium bicarbonate infusions or mucomyst is weak.

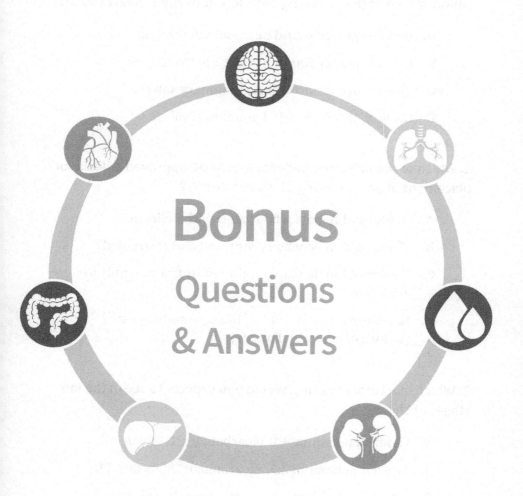

Bonus
Questions
& Answers

Bonus questions:

1. You are auscultating a 74-year-old patient's heart and note a S_4 sound. Which of the following best describes the S_4 heart sound?

    A. Low-frequency sound heard late in diastole

    B. Low-frequency sound heard early in diastole

    C. Closure of the aortic and pulmonary valves

    D. Closure of the tricuspid and mitral valves

2. Which of the following patients meet CDC approved criteria for placement of an indwelling bladder catheter?

    A. 68-year-old female who is alert with delirium

    B. 85-year-old male who is confused and restrained

    C. 72-year-old male with a right femur fracture able to ambulate

    D. 42-year-old female, end-of-life care status post rupture of a cerebral aneurysm

3. Which laboratory findings would you expects to see in the late stages of shock?

    A. Venous potassium 3.1, bicarbonate 32, lactate 1.3

    B. Arterial potassium 3.9, bicarbonate 28, lactate 2.0

    C. Arterial potassium 5.1, bicarbonate 22, lactate 1.9

    D. Venous potassium 6.2, bicarbonate 12, lactate 4.5

4. Which anatomical structure in the kidneys is responsible for the secretion of renin?

    A. Adrenal medulla

    B. Adrenal cortex

    C. Bowman's capsule

    D. Juxtaglomerular cells

5. A 76-year-old patient with end-stage heart failure has decided that he does not want to be resuscitated. Which of the following statements indicates he is accepting & preparing for end of life?

    A. "I wish I would have done more with my life"

    B. "If I could live long enough to watch my grandchildren graduate from college, I would feel complete"

    C. "I feel I have done all the talking I need to do"

    D. "I am not going to bother taking these medications anymore, they don't help"

6. A patient is admitted after collapsing in church at his wife's funeral. He has a history of renal transplant 10 years ago and is currently on tacrolimus (ProGraf), mycophenolate (CellCept), and prednisone (Deltasone). The patient complains of fatigue, nausea, and abdominal pain; vital signs show HR 150 and BP 75/40 (51). The patient is most likely experiencing:

    A. Transplant rejection

    B. Secondary adrenal insufficiency

    C. Myxedema coma

    D. Broken heart syndrome

7. A 51-year-old male is admitted with acute GI bleeding. Which of the following interventions should take priority?

    A. Vasopressor infusion

    B. Intravascular volume replacement

    C. Correction of coagulopathy

    D. Endoscopic intervention

8. A 33-year-old female, who just delivered twins, is transferred to the PCU for bleeding and has received 3 units of packed red blood cells. You should anticipate which of the following interventions next?

    A. Calcium Gluconate and potassium chloride administration

    B. Acetaminophen and diphenhydramine administration

    C. Furosemide 20 mg IV

    D. Fresh frozen plasma and platelets transfusions

9. The bedside monitor alarms demonstrating an irregular, narrow complex tachycardia at a rate of 180. The patient denies chest pain and has a strong palpable pulse, BP is 100/54 (69). Which of the following medication orders is most appropriate?

    A. Magnesium Sulfate 2 Grams IV push x 1

    B. Adenosine 6 mg rapid IV push

    C. Digoxin 0.125 mg IV x 1

    D. Amiodarone 150 mg IV bolus over 10 minutes

10. A patient is admitted to the PCU with an epidural hematoma after a motorcycle collision. This type of intracranial bleeding is:

    A. Venous in origin and is associated with a compound skull fracture

    B. Venous in origin and is associated with a basilar skull fracture

    C. Arterial in origin and is associated with a depressed skull fracture

    D. Arterial in origin and is associated with a linear skull fracture

Bonus questions answers with rationale

1. A. Low-frequency sound heard late in diastole. The S_4 heart sound occurs immediately prior to the first heart sound and is a low-frequency sound heard late in diastole. It is also referred to as a pre-systolic gallop. The S_4 is a vibratory sound caused during forceful atrial contraction of blood into a stiff, non-compliant ventricle. Patients with left ventricular hypertrophy and aortic stenosis often have a S_4 heart sound.

2. D. 42-year-old female, end-of-life care status post rupture of a cerebral aneurysm. CDC approved indications for indwelling urinary catheterization include: strict I&O, immobility, select surgical procedures, perineal or sacral wounds, urinary retention/obstruction, and end-of-life care.

3. D. Venous potassium 6.2, bicarbonate 12, lactate 4.5. During late stages of shock, oxygen rich blood is diverted from the peripheral circulation and is shunted to the vital organs. This poor tissue perfusion leads to anaerobic metabolism, ischemia, and eventually cellular death. Inadequate blood flow to the kidneys results in poor filtration and retention of potassium and inability to regulate bicarbonate. This results in an increase in potassium and lactic acid and a decrease in bicarbonate.

4. D. Juxtaglomerular cells. The juxtaglomerular apparatus secretes renin in response to reduced glomerular filtration pressure.

5. C. "I feel I have done all the talking I need to do". Patients who have lived with heart failure have often had time to prepare for end of life. Acknowledging that he has worked through the situation and is done talking is a good indicator that the patient is ready. Denial, regret, or hope for a future, while normal responses and stages of grief, do not indicate acceptance of death.

6. **B. Secondary adrenal insufficiency.** In the presence of long term steroid use, additional stress can overwhelm the hypothalamic-pituitary-adrenal system. Adrenal insufficiency can be life threatening, so needs to be considered, particularly in patients with steroid use. Transplant rejection would give flu-like symptoms, fever, decreased urine output, and pain. Myxedema coma may also cause hypotension but is more likely to be accompanied by bradycardia rather than tachycardia. Broken heart syndrome, or Takotsubo cardiomyopathy, causes chest pain and shortness of breath.

7. **B. Intravascular volume replacement.** Rapid correction of hypovolemia is needed to prevent end organ hypoperfusion. Initial volume resuscitation should be accomplished with crystalloids, then, depending on clinical status and laboratory values, a transfusion of red blood cells may be necessary. Efforts to treat coagulopathy occur after initial fluid resuscitation. Vasopressors or endoscopy may be used to treat underlying esophageal varices, but not as an initial intervention.

8. **D. Fresh frozen plasma and platelets infusions.** Packed red blood cells are beneficial for oxygenating blood, but do not include all the clotting factors of whole blood. When transfusing large volumes of packed RBC's, an infusion of fresh frozen plasma and platelets are also required, otherwise hemorrhage will continue without adequate clotting factors available. Calcium will need to be replaced, as banked red blood cells use citrate to prevent the blood from clotting. Calcium binds with this citrate, causing hypocalcemia. Potassium levels should not become depleted with blood transfusions therefore would not require repletion. Acetaminophen and diphenhydramine would only be administered if there were a transfusion reaction.

Furosemide is not typically given with massive transfusion, unless pulmonary edema was of serious concern.

9. **D. Amiodarone 150 mg IV bolus over 10 minutes.** Magnesium Sulfate is appropriate treatment for Torsades de Pointes especially in the setting of hypomagnesemia. The patient is stable with a pulse and blood pressure. Amiodarone is an appropriate next step. Adenosine would not be indicated as the rhythm is irregular indicating atrial fibrillation. Digoxin is not appropriate as an anti-arrhythmic in this first step.

10. **D. Arterial in origin and is associated with a linear skull fracture.** An epidural hematoma develops from bleeding into the space between the dura mater and the periosteum. Epidural hematomas account for roughly a quarter of all hematomas. More than 85% are arterial in origin and are most commonly associated with linear skull fractures, which cross over major blood vessels.

You can do it!

About the author...

Nicole Kupchik has practiced as a Critical Care nurse for over twenty years. She obtained a Nursing Degree from Purdue University in 1993 and a Master of Nursing from the University of Washington in 2008.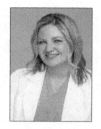

Nicole's nursing career began in the Chicago area. From 1995 to 1998, she journeyed across the United States as a traveling nurse, after which she landed in Seattle. Her first job in Seattle was in the Cardiothoracic Intensive Care Unit (5 SE) at the University of Washington. In 2001, she began working at Harborview Medical Center—a change that spurred an interest in resuscitation.

Shortly thereafter, Nicole was part of a multidisciplinary team that was one of the first in the United States to implement therapeutic hypothermia after cardiac arrest. As part of this effort, Nicole was responsible for protocol development and has published numerous papers on this topic.

In 2008, Nicole led a team that implemented a formalized Sepsis program at Harborview Medical Center. The program resulted in a reduction in mortality, hospital length of stay and a significant cost avoidance. She collaborated with IT specialists to develop innovative methods to electronically screen hospitalized patients in acute care units for sepsis. For this work, the program was awarded two Patient Safety & Clinical Leadership awards.

In 2002, Nicole obtained certification as a CCRN®. She admittedly attended three certification review courses before finally taking the exam! Once she passed the exam she questioned why she hesitated and lacked confidence to sit the exam. Shortly thereafter, Nicole began teaching segments of CCRN® certification review courses at her hospital. In 2006, she started co-teaching courses nationally.

Currently, she works as a staff nurse at Harborview Medical Center in Seattle, WA. She holds certification as a CCNS®, CCRN®, PCCN® & CMC®. In 2013, Nicole founded Nicole Kupchik Consulting & Education. She frequently teaches review courses nationally.

Today her courses are well attended and often sell out! Her wit and sense of humor make the course interesting & entertaining. Nicole has a gift of being able to break information down in a way that is really easy to understand. She hopes to instill confidence in attendees that they can do it!

OTHER BOOKS BY NICOLE KUPCHIK

Ace the CCRN®: You can do it! Study Guide
Ace the CCRN®: You can do it! Practice Review Questions
Ace the PCCN®: You can do it! Study Guide

TO CONTACT NICOLE:

nicole@nicolekupchikconsulting.com

www.nicolekupchikconsulting.com

Nicole Kupchik Consulting and Education

Made in the USA
Middletown, DE
13 November 2020

23786608R00149